MW01442181

DR. SEBI ALKALINE DIET

A Practical Detox & Dieting Strategy to Reverse Disease, Cleanse the Liver & Live Healthy

Kat Marie-Claire

©2019

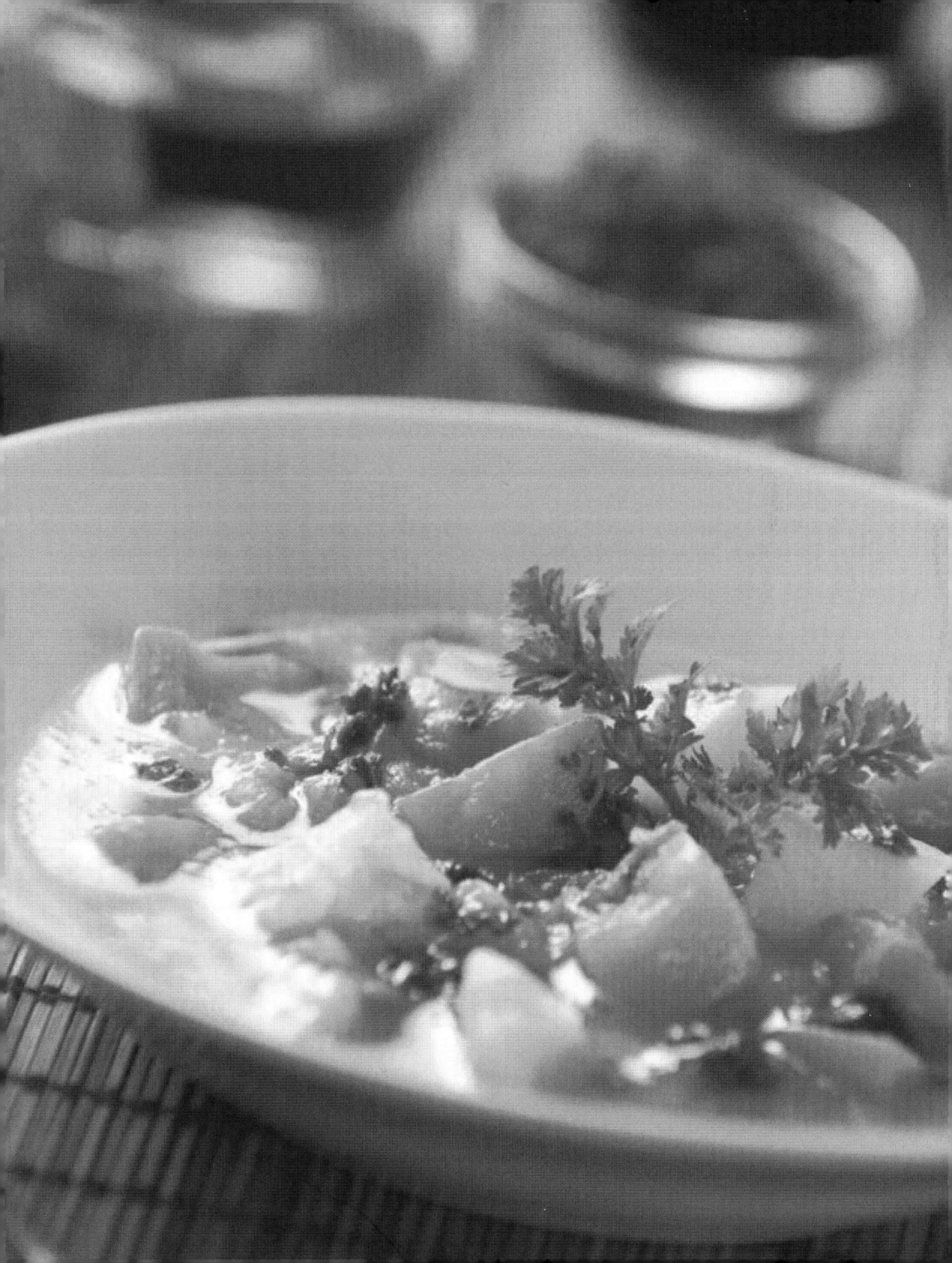

Kat Marie-Claire

COPYRIGHT ©2019

All rights reserved. Except as permitted under the U.S. Copyright Act of 1976, the scanning, uploading and distribution of this book via the internet or via any other means without the express permission of the author is illegal and punishable by law. Please purchase only authorized electronic and paperback editions, and do not participate in, or encourage electronic piracy of copyrighted material.

This publication is designed to provide competent and reliable information regarding the subject matter covered. However, it is sold with the understanding that the author is not engaged in rendering professional or nutritional advice. Laws and practices often vary from state to state and country to country and if medical or other expert assistance is required, the services of a professional should be sought. The author specifically disclaims any liability that is incurred from the use or application of the contents of this book.

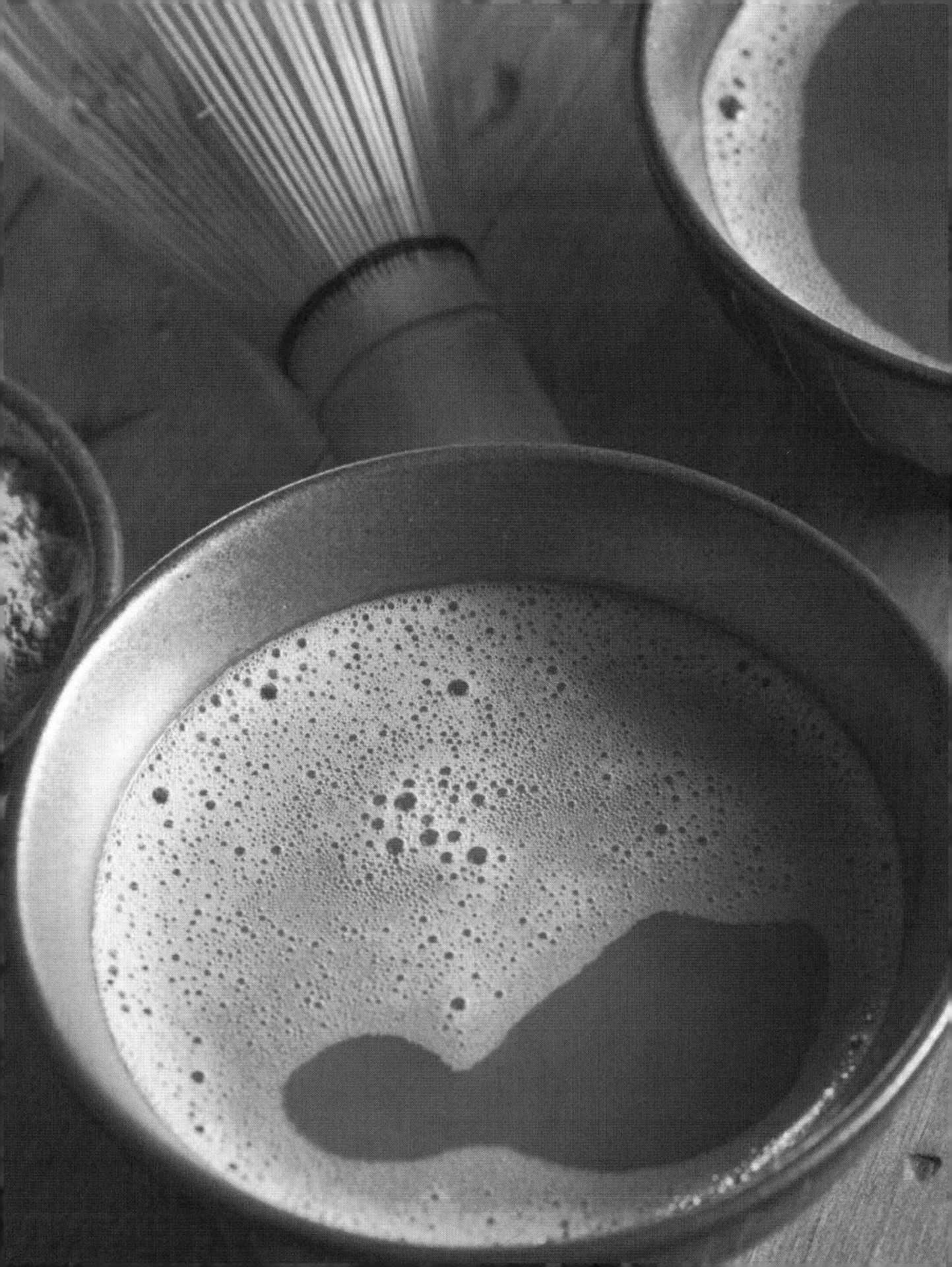

CONTENTS

ABOUT THIS BOOK 11

INTRODUCTION 12

CHAPTER 1 13

WHY DR. SEBI'S DIET? 13

The Alkaline Scale 13

CHAPTER 2 17

ABOUT DR. SEBI 17

How Is Dr. Sebi Diet Different From Other Alkaline Diets 19
3 Principles Of Dr. Sebi Alkaline Diet 20

CHAPTER 3 21

DR. SEBI ALKALINE FOODS 21

How To Gradually Switch To The Dr. Sebi Alkaline Diet 21
Dr. Sebi Food List 23
Dr. Sebi-Approved Vegetables 23
Dr. Sebi-Approved Fruits 24
Dr. Sebi-Approved Spices And Seasonings 25
Alkaline Grains 25
Alkaline Sugars And Sweeteners 25
Dr. Sebi-Approved Herbal Teas 25

CHAPTER 4 27

HYBRID FOODS 27

Why Are Hybrid Foods Excluded From Dr. Sebi Diet? 27

CHAPTER 5 31

YES FOODS, NO FOODS 31

CHAPTER 6 43

CAN DISEASE BE SLOWED DOWN OR REVERSED WITH A DIET? 43

Managing Your Condition With A Diet 43
Benefits Of A Healthy Diet 44

CHAPTER 7 47

HEALTH CONDITIONS DR. SEBI DIET CAN HEAL 47

CHAPTER 8 51

DIABETES 51

The Diabetes Epidemic 51
Main Causes Of Diabetes 53

CHAPTER 9 55
REVERSING FULL-BLOWN DIABETES WITH A LIFESTYLE CHANGE 55
CHAPTER 10 57
HOW TO REVERSE DIABETES THE DR. SEBI WAY 57
The Complete List Of Dr. Sebi-Recommended Herbs 59
3 Herbs Dr. Sebi Particularly Recommended For Diabetes 60
CHAPTER 11 63
DR. SEBI ALKALINE RECIPES 63
Breakfast 63
SPELT WAFFLE 63
BLUEBERRY CAKE 63
BANANA NUT MUFFINS 64
TEFF PORRIDGE 64
QUINOA PORRIDGE WITH APPLE 64
VEGETABLE OMELET 65
HERBAL BREAD 65
SPELT GRANOLA 66
KAMUT PORRIDGE 66
BLUEBERRY SPELT PANCAKES 67
APPLE QUINOA PORRIDGE 67
KAMUT PUFFS 68
Basics 69
CHEESE 69
HEMP MILK 69
WALNUT MILK 69
TAHINI PASTE 70
PIZZA CRUST 70
CUCUMBER PICKLE 70
AQUAFABA 71
SPICY OIL 71
WHIPPED CREAM 71
BLACKBERRY JAM 72
GINGER TEA 72
Lunch 73
WATERCRESS SALAD 73

WILD RICE & MUSHROOMS 73
ZUCCHINI QUINOA SALAD 74
KAMUT PATTIES 74
KALE SALAD 75
MUSHROOM SOUP 75
CHICKPEAS SALAD 76
CUCUMBER MUSHROOM SALAD 76
TACOS 77
MACARONI & CHEESE 77
QUINOA RICE 78
AMARANTH WITH PEARS 78
GARBANZO BEAN BURGER 79
GAZPACHO SOUP 79
SPAGHETTI SQUASH 80
Snacks 81
AMARANTH CRACKERS 81
ONION RINGS 81
CHICKPEA FRENCH FRIES 82
CHICKPEA PATTIES 82
BAKED NUTS 83
TAHINI PRALINE 83
ENERGY BALLS 83
BAKED KALE CHIPS 84
CHIPS 84
DATES BALL 85
SWEETENED CHICKPEAS 85
RAISIN COOKIES 85
Desserts 87
MANGO COCONUT SHERBET 87
BANANA WALNUT ICE CREAM 87
BLUEBERRY CHICKPEA CAKE 87
WALNUT DATE NOG 88
CITRUS FRUIT SALAD 88
MANGO CHEESECAKE 89
STRAWBERRY SORBET 89

Strawberry Ice Cream 90
Applesauce 90
Avocado Yoghurt Sauce 91
Dinner 92
Spelt Bread 92
Chayote Mushroom Soup 92
Kale With Pepper 93
Zucchini Pasta 93
Chickpeas Cornbread 93
Zucchini Bread 94
Chickpea Soup 94
Strawberry Salad 95
Mashed Squash 95
Quinoa Avocado Salad 96
Macaroni & Cheese 96
Sautéed Greens 97
Veggie Quinoa 97
Dips & Sauces 98
Mayonnaise 98
Mango Salsa 98
Guacamole 98
Cucumber Dressing 99
Salsa Verde 99
Avocado Sauce 99
Hummus 100
BBQ Sauce 100
Mango Dressing 100
Tomato Sauce 101
Coleslaw 101
Hot Sauce 102
Smoothies 103
Strawberry Banana Smoothie 103
Green Monster Smoothie 103
Cucumber Coconut Smoothie 104
Apple Smoothie 104

BERRY WALNUT SMOOTHIE 105
WATERMELON SMOOTHIE 105
PEACH BERRY SMOOTHIE 106
CUCUMBER TOMATO SMOOTHIE 106
DETOX GREEN SMOOTHIE 106
PEAR SMOOTHIE 107
CUCUMBER WATERMELON SMOOTHIE 107
ORANGE BERRY SMOOTHIE 107
BANANA GINGER SMOOTHIE 108
PAPAYA SMOOTHIE 108
QUINOA PEAR SMOOTHIE 108

Dr. Sebi

ABOUT THIS BOOK

The concept of alkaline and acidic foods has been known since the middle of the 19th century. Dr. Sebi took this concept a step further and developed a dietary protocol that includes fasting and herbal remedies.

His version of the alkaline diet is renowned for eliminating toxic waste by alkalizing the blood. Dr. Sebi's diet is based on a shortlist of approved foods and a long list of supplements. Although this may not be the easiest of the diets, it has helped many people who were written off by conventional medicine.

In this guide, we take a look at the diet, approved foods, herbs and regimen of the Dr. Sebi alkaline diet.

<u>Specifically, you'll learn</u>
–Understanding the Dr. Sebi alkaline diet
–How does Dr. Sebi alkaline diet work?
–Pros and cons of the diet
–Does science support Dr. Sebi alkaline diet?
–How is Dr. Sebi diet different from the alkaline diet?
–Why are hybrid foods unhealthy?
–How to gradually switch to Dr. Sebi alkaline diet?
–Dr. Sebi-approved foods
–How to slow down or reverse disease with Dr. Sebi's diet
–How to reverse pre-diabetes and diabetes Dr. Sebi way
–How to reverse disease with Dr. Sebi diet–Health conditions that can be improved with Dr. Sebi diet
–How to detox and alkalize your body
–Best ways to detox

<u>Also in this book, you'll learn:</u>
- All Dr. SEBI approved foods and herbs and how you can you use it for optimum health
- How to deal with Pre-Diabetes and Diabetes the Dr. Sebi Way and engage your body to heal and recover faster and better
- How to limit non-alkaline foods and prevent other food cravings
- 5 important secrets why going on the Dr. Sebi alkaline diet is good for you
- How Dr. Sebi Alkaline diet Can Help you with reversing disease, weight loss, improved brain and memory function

INTRODUCTION

Although conventional medicine is still skeptical about how beneficial an alkaline diet really is, it's not true that the benefits of the alkaline diet are not supported by scientific studies. There are hundreds of research papers published in scientific journals throughout the world which generally agree that an alkaline diet helps reduce morbidity and mortality from chronic disease. We know that certain foods affect the body's pH levels. Good health requires a healthy pH balance within the body. This is necessary because, to function properly, organs and fluids need a balanced pH level. To understand the importance of an alkaline diet, you have to know why our modern diet is so acidic. Ever since we started practicing agriculture and adopted a settled lifestyle, our diet has been steadily changing. This happened about 10,000 years ago and this period is known as the Agricultural Revolution. Although this seems like a very long time, in an evolutionary sense, this is like something that happened just a few minutes ago.

So, until about 200 years ago, our diet wasn't that bad. Although many of the foods were hybridized, our lifestyle was still not as sedentary as it is today, the environment contained much fewer toxins than it does today, and our diet did not contain processed foods. We ate mainly carbs, vegetables, dairy, and only occasionally, meat. The main sources of sugar were fruits and honey. Foods were minimally processed. Then, the Industrial Revolution changed everything. Ever since, our diet has contained more and more refined grains, unhealthy fats, and sugar. It also became increasingly rich in inflammatory foods. As most of the chronic diseases of civilization are diet-related, it's obvious that something is very wrong with our eating habits. The life-threatening diseases plaguing the modern world, which can all be slowed down or reversed with a healthy diet, are cardiovascular disease, stroke, cancer, autoimmune disorders, obesity, diabetes, depression, etc.

Chapter 1

Why Dr. Sebi's Diet?

Compared to what we eat today, the diet of 200 or more years ago was very alkaline. It was based on whole grains, little meat, and organic fruits and vegetables. Combined, these foods produced a "net alkaline effect." The human body is an amazing organism and the reason we have as a species survived for so long is that our body has means of self-repair. This includes maintaining good pH levels regardless of what we eat.

The Alkaline Scale

The pH scale runs from 0 to 14. While 0 is acidic, 14 is alkaline or basic; and the midpoint, 7 is neutral. Ideally, pure water is on a scale of pH 7. Ideally, we should try to maintain a pH level of around 7.4. However, not all our organs and fluids require the same acidity level. For example, to be able to break down food, our stomach needs to be acidic (around 4 pH). Some other organs require even higher acidity, e.g. duodenum is 7-8.5, small and large intestine 4-7, etc. So organs that are involved with food processing have high acidity. On the other hand, blood is usually neutral.

When the pH level of a particular organ or system becomes too high or too low, this affects our health in many ways. For instance, the inside of your stomach is lined with a thick layer of mucus that protects it from being destroyed by your stomach's natural acidity. On the other hand, the small intestine has alkaline bile released into it which offers protection from the stomach acidity.

Proper pH is essential for good health and an extreme imbalance (either too much or not enough of acidity) can be fatal. In the absence of balance, you develop either acidosis or alkalosis. Acidosis is characterized by high acidity. There are several different types of acidosis: respiratory, metabolic, renal (kidneys), and lactic acidosis. Symptoms include fatigue, lethargy, confusion, and shortness of breath. Furthermore, metabolic acidosis is the commonly associated with the alkaline diet, but this condition can also be the result of kidney disease or dehydration. Besides, this type of acidosis increases your risk of developing cardiovascular disease, diabetes, insulin resistance, and kidney stones. Diet-induced metabolic acidosis is the consequence of eating too much meat, and not enough fruits and vegetables.

On the other hand, alkalosis is also a potentially dangerous health condition. It occurs when blood or bodily fluids become extremely alkaline. It's a condition that can be caused by low oxygen levels, a sudden loss of electrolytes or lung or liver disease. Symptoms include confusion, lightheadedness, and muscle spasm, seizure, tingling in the extremities and face, and respiratory problems.

Background

Most of us have, at some stage, tried following a particular diet. This was not necessarily for weight management. As we are, generally, better informed today than we were twenty years ago, we have also become more health-conscious. This is why most diets focus on improving one's health. However, there is a problem. What makes dieting difficult in this day and age is that there is a lot of conflicting information about what you should or shouldn't eat. To complicate things further, all the diets claim to be healthy. Even nutritionists often can't agree on what the healthiest diet is.

Why are there so many different healthy diets and are they really all healthy? The reason all the new diets claim to be healthy is that with the scientific advancements of the 20th century, we've become aware of the importance of nutrition. We now know how different types of fats affect our body and what foods we can use to reverse or at least slow down certain diseases. So, most of the new diets are created with these scientific discoveries in mind and they really are healthy.

However, this begs a million-dollar-question: Healthy for whom?

Our nutritional needs depend on many things, e.g. age, occupation, gender, overall health, etc. A diet suitable for an athlete is very different from the one recommended to a cancer patient. While an athlete needs the energy to boost his physical performance, a cancer patient needs foods that support the immune system and help with detoxification. In other words, food that would benefit an athlete could kill a cancer patient or a diabetic.

Besides, we are all different. A Paleo diet comes with many health benefits, but so does a vegetarian diet. We all have certain preferences (eg you don't eat meat), underlying health conditions (eg an allergy) or nutritional requirements (eg you are a breastfeeding woman) that make certain foods agree with us or not. A diet that one person can benefit from, could make another person ill. The alkaline diet revolves around foods that help maintain an optimal pH level in the body. These foods are mainly vegetables, ideally raw. However, this is not a vegan diet. Eating alkaline foods is not enough. You also need to eliminate all acid-forming foods.

An alkaline diet consists of two steps:
- You eat as many vegetables as possible
- You limit or eliminate foods that, once ingested, contribute to fermentation

On the alkaline diet, you make sure that 70-80% of the foods you eat are vegetables, ideally raw. The remaining 20-30% of your diet should revolve around whole grains, lean protein, healthy oils, and nuts & seeds.

Animal products should be either eliminated or limited to 5%.

Chapter 2

About Dr. Sebi

Who is Dr. Sebi?

Alfonso Darrington Bowman (1933-2016), also known as Dr. Sebi, was a Honduran herbalist and healer. He claimed to be able to cure even the most serious diseases with herbs and a special diet. The diet he recommended was based on alkaline foods. Although he called himself Dr. Sebi, Bowman was not a doctor and did not have formal medical training.

Dr. Sebi developed a diet based on the African Bio Mineral Balance theory which he claimed could reverse even the most serious diseases, e.g. AIDS, cancer, diabetes, etc. However, Dr. Sebi did not create the well-known alkaline diet. The concept of alkaline and acidic foods has been known since the middle of the 19-th century. Dr. Sebi took this concept a step further and developed a dietary protocol that includes fasting and herbal remedies. His version of the alkaline diet is renowned for eliminating toxic waste by alkalizing your blood. Dr. Sebi's diet is based on a short list of approved foods and a long list of supplements. Although this may not be the easiest of the diets, it has helped many people who were written off by conventional medicine. For this diet to be sustainable, it should be consistently followed for the rest of your life.

Dr. Sebi was a controversial figure and a lot of information about his life is missing from his biography. Still, his healing method became very popular and many people claim Dr. Sebi alkaline diet helped them recover their vitality and health.

HISTORY
Dr. Sebi's first experience with herbalism came from watching his grandmother. Later, when conventional medicine couldn't help him cure his asthma, diabetes, and impotency, he visited a herbalist in Mexico, who he claimed managed to help him with his health problems. This is when he took herbalism seriously. Over time, he

opened a herbal healing practice in New York and started another practice in a village of Usha in Honduras that he called the USHA Research Institute.

Among his clients were some well-known celebrities, eg John Travolta, Lisa Lopes, Eddie Murphy, Michael Jackson, and Steven Seagal. However, after being sued in New York, he relocated to LA in California.

In 1987, New York City sued him for practicing medicine without a license. Although he was acquitted, he was later sued by the New York Attorney General for claiming he could cure untreatable diseases such as AIDS, cancer, leukemia, lupus, etc. He was forbidden to make therapeutic claims for his products.

In 2016, Dr. Sebi was taken into custody for money laundering and held for many weeks in a Honduran prison. By the time police officials realized how sick he was and decided to transfer him to a hospital, it was too late. He died en route to the hospital due to complications of pneumonia. Dr. Sebi did not consider himself an African Honduran, but an African in Honduras. At the time of his death, he had 17 children. According to his website, Dr. Sebi developed his unique methodology for healing the human body after extensively studying herbs in North America, Central and South America, Africa, and the Caribbean.

How Is Dr. Sebi Diet Different From Other Alkaline Diets

The concept of the alkaline diet is not a new one. It's been known since the middle of the 19-th century. Although some of the aspects of the alkaline diet were used by many nutritionists and holistic practitioners, the alkaline diet became popular relatively recently.

It was during the 1990s, that some nutritionists started suggesting a 100% alkaline diet. Dr. Sebi took this a step further. He developed a diet that revolved around maintaining vitality by using the "African Bio Mineral Balance". Dr. Sebi referred to his method as either the African Bio-mineral balance or the African Bio Balance. The African Bio-mineral Balance remedy consists of 102 minerals that support electrical activity and overall vitality of the body. This therapeutic approach addresses disease on two levels. It first cleanses the body of acidity. This step relies heavily on herbs that clean the body's cells on both the cellular and intra-cellular level. The next step is to revitalize cells by supplying minerals that have been lost through the consumption of acidic foods.

Unfortunately, 90% of the modern diet is based on acidic foods, e.g. meat, dairy, processed foods as well as GMO and hybridized foods. Eating these foods will acidify the body and unbalance the alkalinity of the blood. The reason Dr. Sebi insisted on unhybridized fruits and vegetables is that such foods have an alkaline base. They were designed by nature to provide a human body with all it needs for optimal health. Dr. Sebi developed his approach to health on the assumption that disease can only exist in an acidic environment. The body works non-stop to maintain a 7.4 pH level in the blood. When you eat a balanced diet, your body is perfectly capable of maintaining this level of acidity. However, the modern diet is very unbalanced. It is based on carbs, meat, sugar, and junk food which are all very acidic and which is why our body needs help to maintain homeostasis.

Some of the cleansing herbs Dr. Sebi used in his alkaline diet are burdock root, sarsaparilla, and dandelion, which clean the blood and the liver. Dr. Sebi diet revolves around three principles that are simple to follow and that everyone can easily fit into their lifestyle, no matter how hectic or unusual.

3 Principles of Dr. Sebi Alkaline Diet

1. **Food list**

Eat only the foods that are on the Dr. Sebi food list. The list is very specific (and restrictive) and excludes many nutritious foods. Dr. Sebi believed strongly in natural foods and insisted one should stay away from hybridized fruits and vegetables (i.e. plants produced by unnatural cross-pollination). He was adamant that these foods have their genetic structure, electrical composition, and pH balance changed and are therefore not suitable for human consumption.

2. **Springwater**

Drinking about 4 liters of water a day is necessary partly because 70% of our body is water, and partly because water helps with the detoxification process. Waste that remains in the body for too long (eg when you are constipated) becomes toxic. Water also helps with the absorption of nutrients. This is why many of the herbs Dr. Sebi recommends are diuretics that increase urination and so help remove toxins from the body. Springwater may not be easy to come by nowadays but it provides the best hydration.

3. **No microwaving**

Dr. Sebi considered food prepared in microwave unhealthy and recommended the use of a stove or oven for heating or cooking your meals. An ideal solution would be eating raw foods whenever possible. Dr. Sebi believed that with the alkaline diet it's possible to both prevent and cure disease. According to him, the disease is a result of mucus build-up in an area of your body. For example, a build-up of mucus in the lungs causes pneumonia, while excess mucus in the pancreas leads to diabetes, etc. Dr. Sebi argued that diseases cannot exist in an alkaline environment and only occur when your body becomes too acidic. He believed that by strictly following his diet and using the prescribed supplements, it's possible to restore your body's ideal pH levels and get rid of the accumulated toxins.

Dr. Sebi alkaline diet comprises of a list of approved fruits, vegetables, grains, seeds, herbs, nuts and oils. He claimed that for your body to heal itself, and stay healthy, you must follow the diet consistently for the rest of your life.

Chapter 3

DR. SEBI ALKALINE FOODS

Alkaline foods are some of the healthiest foods there are, and they are particularly recommended to those suffering from frequent colds because of the suppressed immune system, headaches, low energy, anxiety, and benign breast and ovarian cysts. The foods that are known to contribute to acid and that we usually eat a lot of are red meat, pasta, sweets, and dairy. Changing a diet, especially if it is supposed to be a drastic change, is not easy. To improve your health, you have to find a way of reducing the acid load and adopting healthier eating habits.

How to Gradually Switch to the Dr. Sebi Alkaline Diet
Many people don't enjoy dieting but the best results are achieved when the desire to change your eating habits is self-imposed, rather than suggested by someone else, e.g. doctor, colleague, partner, etc.

It's best to proceed slowly and set a goal, e.g. to lower your cholesterol levels. However, what seems to be even more difficult from changing a diet is maintaining it. Most diets are to a certain degree restrictive and although most people usually stick to a diet for a while, i.e. until they've achieved their goals, e.g. to lose a certain amount of weight, what everyone finds very difficult is sticking to a new dietary regimen for extended periods.

One of the methods for a "smooth transition" is that, before going on a diet, you start eating healthy. If you're eating habits are not that bad this will be relatively easy, but if you live on junk food, then you'll struggle. For example, to prepare yourself for adopting the alkaline diet, you may gradually start to increase the quantity of plant-based foods in your meals.

Another way of tricking your body into eating healthy foods is a method called "crowding out". It's very simple, instead of giving up on unhealthy foods; you simply add healthy foods to your diet.

For example, you eat meat but you also have a big salad with every meal. Or, you first eat healthy foods and then unhealthy ones, e.g. you first eat your veggies, and only then you fill your plate with meat or dairy. The idea is that by the time you start eating meat, you already feel full which means you will eat less meat than you would have otherwise. Or, if you have a sweet tooth and can't give up desserts, first have some fruits and only then have a piece of cake. Ideally, as fruits are full of fiber, they will easily fill you up so you won't have space for pudding.

What are the benefits of crowding out? They boil down to this:
— **Nutrients**
Your body will get all the nutrients it needs from the healthy foods (those you eat first) even if your diet is generally unhealthy.
— **Food preferences**
The more you eat healthy foods, the greater the chance you'll get used to them and hopefully start preferring them to unhealthy foods.
— **Cravings**
If your main problem with following a healthy diet is craving for unhealthy foods, you should know that craving usually means you lack certain nutrients. So, if you eat nutrient-dense foods, chances are you will get all the nutrients you need and will stop craving.

Dr. Colleen Huber, the founder of *Nature Works Best Medical Clinic,* believes we should take cravings seriously. According to her, cravings are a sign of mild malnutrition. This phenomenon is wide-spread even in developed countries. However, cravings are easy to cure if you replace the foods you crave with nutritious foods. For example:
- If you crave **chocolate**, what you need is magnesium and you can get it from raw nuts and seeds, and fruits
- If you crave **bread**, what you need is nitrogen which can be found in protein-rich foods, e.g. nuts and beans
- If you crave **simple carbs** such as bread and pasta, what your body needs is the amino acid tryptophan. This acid is essential for the production of the "feel-good" hormone *serotonin*. So, if you are often in a bad mood, you may be subconsciously trying to cheer yourself up by craving high-carb foods.

Dr. Sebi

To make the transition to a healthy diet easier, take a lot of liquids, eg water, herbal teas, soups, etc. These are not only filling and will help you feel full even if you are hungry but will make it easier to keep your organs hydrated.

Dr. Sebi Food List

The body produces all the acid it needs, so when your urine pH levels are high, it means that your body is trying to rid itself of excess acid. This excess acid gets into your organs through acidic foods and beverages. Fortunately, your body continually tries to maintain balance and will not tolerate the surplus of acid so it gets rid of it. However, if you continually, over many months and years, consume very acidic foods, your kidneys and lungs will eventually become unable to process the surplus and you'll develop acidosis.

Most of the surplus of acids come from proteins. An easy solution to this problem, if you can't avoid or reduce protein, is to simply eat more alkaline foods (ie fruits and vegetables). That way, alkaline foods will reduce acid levels. However, the trouble is that the modern diet contains too many neutral foods, eg starches, fats, and sugar, which are unable to compensate for an acid load.

Dr. Sebi-approved food list is what your diet should focus on if you want to reap the benefits of the alkaline lifestyle. Although many nutritious foods are missing from this list, and many of the foods listed may not be available where you live, it's easy to prepare tasty and varied meals even with only some of the foods from this list.

Dr. Sebi-approved vegetables
- Olives
- Wakame
- Zucchini
- Wild Arugula
- Cucumber
- Mushrooms (but not Shitake)
- Squash
- Onions
- Garbanzo Beans
- Cherry and Plum Tomato
- Tomatillo

- Nori
- Turnip Greens
- Amaranth
- Kale
- Okra
- Watercress
- Dandelion Greens
- Chayote
- Arame
- Lettuce (but not iceberg)
- Bell Pepper
- Avocado

Dr. Sebi-approved fruits

- Cantaloupe
- Bananas
- Prickly Pear
- Peaches
- Soursoups
- Limes
- Cherries
- Plums
- Berries
- Tamarind
- Rasins
- Papayas
- Soft Jelly Coconuts
- Currants
- Apples
- Pears
- Dates
- Figs
- Prunes
- Orange
- Mango

Dr. Sebi

- Grapes
- Melons

Dr. Sebi-approved spices and seasonings
- Oregano
- Cloves
- Tarragon
- Pure Sea Salt
- Powdered Granulated Seaweed
- Cayenne
- Habanero
- Sage
- Sweet Basil
- Dill
- Basil
- Achiote
- Savory
- Thyme
- Onion Powder
- Bay Leaf

Alkaline Grains
- Kamut
- Rye
- Quinoa
- Wild Rice
- Amaranth
- Spelt
- Fonio

Alkaline Sugars and Sweeteners
- Agave Syrup from cactus
- Date Sugar from dried dates

Dr. Sebi-Approved Herbal Teas

Kat Marie-Claire

- Fennel
- Elderberry
- Chamomile
- Red Raspberry
- Tila
- Ginger
- Burdock

Chapter 4

HYBRID FOODS

Why Are Hybrid Foods Excluded From Dr. Sebi Diet?

Hybridization and crossbreeding started when men decided to get the best out of different species of plants or animals. This was deemed necessary for many reasons, e.g.

- New animal species are easier to breed or manage, or they give more milk, wool or meat
- New plant species give produce with thinner skin, better taste, or bigger size
- Hybridized species are more resistant to drought, frost or disease

However, on the downside, the new species often have a very negative effect on the environment, eg they may need much more resources (food or water) than the native species. Or, they are very "nutrient-hungry" and deplete the soil of all the minerals so nothing can grow on such land for many years and the area becomes desert-like. Or, hybridized species replace indigenous species that are more beneficial for local wildlife, etc.

Unfortunately, ever since the Agricultural Revolution 10,000 years ago, people have been regularly hybridizing both plant and animal species. This practice intensified in the last 100 years so almost all the foods we eat have at some stage been hybridized. Some have been with us for so long that we don't realize they never existed in their original state, eg potatoes. Other hybrids are more recent, e.g. boysenberries (a hybrid of raspberries and blackberries), broccolini, cantaloupe, etc.

As a seed of a fruit or vegetable is its "life", the easiest way to find out is a species is hybridized is if it has no seed, e.g. seedless apples, grapes, citrus fruit, watermelons, etc. However, many hybridized species do have the seed (e.g. tomatoes).

Some of the common foods that are hybridized:

- **Fruits**

Apple, grapefruit, Meyer lemon, orange, nectarine, pineapple, etc.

- **Vegetables**

Beets, carrots, corn, potatoes, celery, cauliflower, garlic, most beans and legumes, alfalfa sprouts, etc.

– **Nuts & seeds**

Cashews, peanuts, etc.

– **Grains**

Wheat, rice (brown, white, and "wild" rice), oats, soy, etc.

– **Herbs**

Goldenseal, Ginseng. Echinacea, Chamomile, Aloe Vera, Nutmeg, Comfrey, Peppermint, Spearmint, etc.

– **Seaweeds**

Seaweeds like chlorella, spirulina, and blue-green algae.

The reason Dr. Sebi was so much against hybrid foods is that he believed they lack the essence of life and are high in both sugar and starch. They also lack a proper mineral balance of the "original" species. This means that if your diet is based on hybrid foods (as it probably is) your diet is mineral-deficient.

Hybrid fruits contain more sugar, which is why they taste better but this is bad news for our pancreas. They also contain fewer nutrients compared to natural varieties. So, although many hybrid fruits do contain seeds, avoiding seedless fruits is one of the easiest ways of avoiding unnatural foods in your diet.

Your immune system can be compromised for many reasons, and a combination of acidic foods and nutrient-deficiency is one of them. What's worse, over the years, an inappropriate diet destroys your mucous membrane and paves a way for many health problems.

The mucous membrane is a lining of your digestive, respiratory, and reproductive organs. It protects your internal organs from pathogens and your tissues from dehydration. If it becomes thin or is broken, you become much more vulnerable to disease.

For example, if the mucous membrane of your stomach becomes thin or is damaged eg due to an infection of *Helicobacter pylori*, the stomach acid intended to break down food, will start breaking down your stomach and you will develop gastritis or ulcers.

Dr. Sebi

There are many reasons why the mucous membrane becomes damaged. This partly depends on where in the body it is, but the most common reasons are:

– Lack of hygiene
– Alcohol, tobacco, or drugs abuse
– Acidic foods
– Chemotherapy
– Dehydration
– Depression
– Reduced hormone levels in postmenopausal women
– Immunosuppression
– Infection
– Malnutrition
– Radiation therapy
– Mouth breathing
– Stress

The bottom line is that hybrid foods are not unhealthy and they are certainly not dangerous to eat, but they are unnatural in the sense that they were created by man and not nature.
Are they safe to eat? Look at it this way – most of the foods we eat today have at some point been tampered with by man. So, avoiding hybridized foods is not easy but it can be done.
This is why the list of Dr. Sebi-approved foods is so short. However, since the choice of foods allowed on Dr. Sebi diet is so limited, followers of this diet would deprive themselves of many essential nutrients if they followed this diet without taking the recommended herbal remedies and supplements.
Food is supposed to be a source of nutrition and energy, however, the modern diet is also a source of quite a lot of acid. To balance the pH levels simply avoid or limit acidic foods and increase the intake of alkaline foods. Your body will do the rest.

Kat Marie-Claire

CHAPTER 5
YES FOODS, NO FOODS

Foods You Should Never Eat (and why)

Regardless of the diet you're on, there are usually foods you should eat more of, as well as those you should stay away from. Today, there are dozens of healthy, as well as fad diets, and they all have their "followers."

However, there are some foods everyone should not only stay away from but avoid them like a plague. These foods are more than just unhealthy. Some of them contain so many artificial additives and synthetic chemicals, they are actually dangerous to eat.

Unfortunately, many of these foods are very popular and we eat them all the time. Some of them are even offered by health food shops. When you go through this list, you'll understand why the so-called diseases of civilization are becoming a serious threat to global health.

3 things that most unhealthy foods have in common:
1.   They are popular

Most of these foods are on our table every day. What's even worse, some of them are sold in health food shops as healthy alternatives to sugar, meat or dairy.

2.   They are aggressively marketed

The meat and dairy industries have powerful lobbies that successfully manipulate people into buying foods they shouldn't. Aggressive marketing campaigns and misleading messages have resulted in consumers becoming unable to decide for themselves, but doing what they are told.

3.   They are tasty, cheap, and convenient

What makes giving up these foods so difficult, is that most of them are very tasty (because they are full of flavor additives), cheap (because they are mass-produced from the cheapest ingredients), and convenient (many of them are pre-packed and ready to use, requiring minimum preparation time).

The story of modern agriculture and the stressful sedentary lifestyle we now lead is a long and complicated one and is beyond the scope of this book. Suffice it to say that your diet should be much more than fuel that keeps you going.

A diet can be a source of healing or toxic foods. It can improve or destroy your health. It can boost your mood and performance or contribute to premature aging and chronic disease. So, whatever diet you think is best for you, make sure it's free of the following foods.

24 foods you should never eat (and why):

1. Deep-fried foods

Deep-fried foods are usually very tasty which is why we love them. However, they are cooked in a lot of oil which makes them very fatty. Besides, what makes it even more unhealthy is that such oil is usually reused many times. Avoid or limit these foods if you want to get rid of free radicals, high cholesterol levels, heart disease or acidic diet.

2. Canned foods

All canned foods contain Bisphenol A (BPA). This chemical is used in can lining and has been linked to infertility, obesity, cancer, and other conditions. Whenever possible, choose fresh or frozen foods instead of canned ones.

3. Instant noodles

Instant noodles, just like all other instant foods, are full of preservatives, and color- and flavor additives. Besides, they contain a lot of calories and sodium. If you often eat instant noodles, you risk having a stroke, developing diabetes or succumbing to heart disease.

4. Soft drinks

Soft drinks contain a lot of sugar (about 40 grams per bottle) and if taken regularly will increase your blood sugar levels which can lead to many serious conditions, eg high blood pressure, diabetes, etc.

5.   Margarine

Margarine is based on trans fats. These clog arteries and restrict the flow of blood to the heart. When it first appeared on the market, we were told it was healthier than butter and would protect our hearts. Today, we know this is nonsense. Regular consumption of trans fats increases your risk of developing type 2 diabetes or heart disease.

6.   Fruit juice

Many people start their day with a glass of orange juice. Well, they shouldn't. It takes four oranges to produce a single glass of juice. Although juice is a healthy beverage, unfortunately, all the fiber from the fruit has been discarded. Besides, fruit juice contains almost as much sugar as soft drinks. A better way to start a day would be to eat an orange, not drink a glass of orange juice. That way, you'll get all the vitamins, plus the fiber, and the amount of fructose your liver has to deal with would be minimal.

7.   Soy protein

Most of the soy produced in the US (as well as in some other countries) is genetically modified. The reason GM soy is now farmed is that it is resistant to glyphosate, a weedkiller commonly used in soy farming. A recent Norwegian study found that US-produced soy contains so much of this herbicide, it almost feels like you are eating weedkiller. Glyphosate is linked to many life-threatening conditions, including several types of lymphoma cancer.

While fermented soy products, such as natto, tempeh, and miso soups are perfectly safe to use, you must stay away from edamame, soy milk, and soy protein.

8.   Artificial sweeteners

Artificial sweeteners are found in many sugar-free products, et chewing gums, baked goods, jams, etc. They are also what sugar replacements are based on, eg xylitol, erythritol, isomalt, lactitol, maltitol, mannitol, sorbitol. Although these artificial sweeteners are marketed as natural, they are actually heavily processed and are often produced from GMO ingredients. Long-term use of artificial sweeteners can create an imbalance in your gut flora and contribute to the development of diabetes, gastrointestinal problems, weight gain, etc.

9.   Farmed salmon (Atlantic salmon)
Most people eat salmon because it's high in omega-3 fatty acids. However, farmed salmon available today have considerably lower levels of these healthy fats than the salmon we could buy only five years ago. The most likely reason for this is that salmon is now fed much less nutritious food. Besides, dioxin levels are ten times higher in farmed salmon than in wild salmon. This is bad news because this chemical is linked to cancer, organ damage, and immune system dysfunction.

On top of that, farmed salmon is regularly treated with banned pesticides. To make things even worse, it recently became legal to produce and sell genetically engineered salmon without having to label it as such.

10.   Microwave popcorn
The microwavable bags are lined with perfluorochemicals that make the bags resistant to heat. Unfortunately, these chemicals are linked to cancer. Besides, the fake butter flavoring that's often used in the production of popcorn is known to cause lung disease and inflammation in various organs.

11.   Meat from large-scale farms
All animals raised this way are fed growth hormones, antibiotics, and food grown with chemical pesticides and fertilizers. A recent analysis of chicken meat and feathers discovered traces of banned antibiotics, allergy medications, painkillers, and even arsenic.

12.   Shrimp
Farmed shrimps contain a certain food additive that is used to improve the color of shrimp. This additive has estrogen-like effects that can affect the sperm count in men and increase the risk of breast cancer in women. Besides, ponds where shrimps are raised, are often treated with neurotoxic pesticides known to cause certain neurological problems, eg attention deficit symptoms, impaired memory, etc.

13.   Vegetable oils
Vegetable oils, eg canola, cottonseed, corn or soybean oil, are as bad as margarine. If

you use a lot of oil or eat a lot of deep-fried foods, you will become more vulnerable to certain diseases, eg inflammation, atherosclerosis, certain types of cancer, diabetes, digestive disorders, heart disease, high cholesterol, liver problems, obesity, etc.

14. Salt

Iodine is one of the most essential trace elements our body needs for proper functioning which is why we should use only iodized salt. Salt comes either from underground salt deposits or the sea. Although the natural salt is rich in minerals, by the time it is delivered to shops, it has been processed so much, that none of its original nutrients remain. Besides, salt rich in natural minerals is never white which is why it is bleached (to look clean). After bleaching, various anticaking agents are added to make it free-flowing. Excessive consumption of salt (including the mineral-rich healthy salt) increases the risk of high blood pressure, heart disease, stroke, kidney disease, etc.

15. Fat-free and low-fat milk

When raw milk is pasteurized, it loses a lot of its nutrients. Long-life milk is particularly unhealthy because it first has to be dried at temperatures of about 1000 degrees Centigrade, after which water is added to it. Needless to say, no enzymes or any other nutrients can survive these high temperatures.

People usually choose low-fat or fat-free dairy products because they don't want to gain weight. However, what they don't realize is that when fat is removed, carbs or sugar are added. This is done so that milk would have flavor, otherwise, it would taste like water.

So, fat-free and low-fat milk contains added sugar, which, if you drink a lot of milk, puts you at risk of developing diabetes or heart disease.

16. Seitan

We usually think of seitan as a healthy alternative to meat protein. However, it is simply wheat gluten. This means that even if you are not allergic to gluten but you often eat seitan, you may develop gluten intolerance symptoms. Besides, seitan contains a lot of sodium, over 500 milligrams per 100 grams.

17. Coffee with added flavors

Black coffee has a number of health benefits and can even protect you from certain liver diseases. However, after sugar, whipped cream or powdered milk has been added to it, it becomes a very unhealthy beverage.

It gets even more unhealthy if you add non-dairy liquid creamers based on corn syrup. Black coffee is the healthiest option because although these additives improve the taste of coffee, they also contribute to increased liver fat and some gastrointestinal problems.

18. Agave nectar

Although agave nectar is believed to be the healthiest sugar alternative, it is actually a very unhealthy one. It has the highest fructose content of any sweeteners and is very hard on the liver.

19. Diet soda

The main reason you should avoid diet soda is that it's full of artificial sweeteners. For a number of reasons, these are worse for your health than ordinary sugar. So, if you drink diet soda regularly, you are at a higher risk of developing both cancer and diabetes.

20. Burnt food

Bunt foods should be avoided whenever possible. This is necessary partly because they are more difficult to digest, but especially because they produce cancer-causing chemicals. Burnt meat in particular is very unhealthy. Although many people find charred meat tastier than medium-to-rare, the risk of ingesting carcinogens is not worth the improved taste.

21. Processed meats

Many people can't imagine a sandwich without salami but cured meats are so full of saturated fat, sodium, and preservatives, that if you are into healthy eating, this is one of the first foods you should give up.

22. Non-organic strawberries

Some fruits and vegetables contain so many toxins from pesticides and fertilizers, that they are actually dangerous to eat. One of them is strawberries. Besides the pesticides, the soil on which non-organic strawberries are grown, is often treated with toxic gases. These were initially developed for chemical warfare, but are now used in agriculture. In other words, if you can't afford organic strawberries, stay away from them.

23. Canned green beans

For some reason, U.S.-grown canned green beans are some of the most toxic canned foods there are. This food is treated with some of the most dangerous pesticides and eating just one serving a day, puts you at risk of developing cancer and having other health problems. Besides, all cans are lined with materials that contain Bisphenol A. This is a synthetic estrogen that can create fertility problems for both men and women. Unless you can find fresh or frozen green beans, this is one of the foods you must avoid at all costs.

24. Energy drinks

The reason they are so addictive is that they taste so good. Which they do because they are full of sugar and flavor additives. Long-term use of energy drinks is linked to inflammatory processes, heart disease, and certain neurological problems.

The list of unhealthy foods is much longer but the bottom line is to try and stay away from all processed, instant or foods that don't even look like food. Whenever possible, stick to organically grown fruits and vegetables and grass-fed meat, dairy, and eggs.

Best Disease-Fighting Foods

How successfully you avoid or recover from disease depends on many things but most of all on your diet. Certain foods, or food combinations, are so rich in essential nutrients, you can use them as medicine, not just food.

Perhaps that's what the father of modern medicine, Hippocrates, meant when he said, "Illnesses do not come upon us out of the blue. They are developed from small daily sins against Nature. When enough sins have accumulated, illnesses will suddenly appear."

Kat Marie-Claire

The super-foods listed below may not be available everywhere or may not be available throughout the year, but there are so many of them that regardless of where you live, or which time of the year it is, you are bound to have access to at least some of them.

<u>15 foods that help you fight disease:</u>

1.   Leafy greens
These are spinach, Swiss chard, Bok choy, kale, collard greens, mustard greens, lettuce, arugula, green onions, etc. Dark green leafy vegetables (the darker the better) are some of the most nutritious foods because they are loaded with minerals (eg iron, calcium, potassium, and magnesium) and vitamins (eg vitamins K, C, E, and many of the B vitamins). Try to have some every day.

2.   Broccoli
Because of all the vitamins, minerals, fiber, and antioxidants, broccoli is often referred to as a "nutritional powerhouse." It's best eaten raw because of its high vitamin C content. Regular consumption of broccoli can help you reduce inflammation and avoid certain types of cancer (eg breast, prostate, stomach, colorectal, kidney, and bladder). It also improves the health of your gut and helps the brain recover after a stroke or an injury. It's even more nutritious if combined with tomatoes.

3.   Tomatoes
Tomatoes are a rich source of vitamins, particularly C, A, and K. What's more, a single tomato can provide about 40% of the daily recommended dose of vitamin C. It improves your vision, digestion, and skin. It's rich in lycopene which helps reduce the risk of certain types of cancer, eg prostate, ovarian, lung, and stomach.

4.   Avocado
This fruit is loaded with nutrients and can help improve many health conditions. Avocado is rich in monosaturated fatty acids which you need to maintain a healthy heart and healthy cholesterol and triglyceride levels. It's also loaded with fiber which boosts friendly gut bacteria. Avocado is the food to eat if you undergo chemotherapy

Dr. Sebi

because it helps reduce side effects.

5.   Sweet potato

This starchy root vegetable provides a number of health benefits and is very tasty. Sweet potato is a good source of vitamins C and A, as well as many minerals. This is a powerful anti-inflammatory food that improves gut health, can help you avoid certain types of cancer (eg bladder, colon, stomach, and breast), boosts your brain function, and helps you maintain good vision.

6.   Sauerkraut

Fermentation increases the bioavailability of nutrients which makes sauerkraut even more nutritious than the raw cabbage. It's a rich source of vitamins C and K. It's also rich in minerals, eg calcium, magnesium, folate, iron, potassium, copper, and manganese.

Besides, sauerkraut is what you should eat if you'd like to increase the amount of dietary fiber in your diet and improve digestion and growth of friendly gut bacteria. Sauerkraut should be eaten raw, ie uncooked and unpasteurized, because that way it contains live *Lactobacilli* and is rich in enzymes that inhibit the growth of cancer cells.

7.   Garlic

Garlic is believed to be the best natural antibiotic. It helps prevent or reduce symptoms of many common illnesses, eg cold and flu. It also lowers the high blood pressure, improves cholesterol levels, prevents Alzheimer's and dementia if taken regularly, improves physical performance, and helps with detox. Try to get used to the taste and eat it every day.

8.   Eggs (organic or grass-fed)

An excellent source of protein for vegetarians, eggs are incredibly nutritious. Eggs are rich in vitamins A, B complex, D, E, and K as well as minerals (calcium, zinc, selenium, phosphorous). They are also high in protein and essential amino acids and can help you increase muscle mass, lower blood pressure, and improve eye health. Being very filling, they also help with weight loss.

9.   Olive oil

Cold-pressed olive oil is the best oil there is. It's rich in healthy monosaturated acids that help reduce inflammation, contains a lot of antioxidants that protect you from chronic disease, stroke and heart problems, has anti-cancer properties, relieves rheumathoid arthritis inflammation, and helps fight infections.

10. Blueberries

High in vitamins, minerals, and fiber, blueberries have the highest antioxidant level of all fruits. Regular consumption of these berries is one of the best protection against premature aging and cancer. Blueberries can prevent heart disease, improve cognitive performance, help with urinary tract infections, boost your eye health, and much more. Besides, by keeping your brain sharp, they indirectly protect you against Alzheimer's.

11. Lemon

Lemon is very rich in vitamin C and soluble fiber, a combination that helps protect you against heart disease. It is also efficient protection against kidney stones, anemia, cancer, and various digestive problems. Take it as often as you can.

12. Apples

This popular fruit is so nutrient-dense, that eating them regularly lowers the risk of many diseases. Apples can stabilize blood glucose levels, reduce the risk of diabetes, maintain a healthy cholesterol level, and a healthy heart. Besides, an apple a day will improve your digestion, reduce the risk of certain types of cancer, diabetes, and stroke.

13. Walnuts and almonds

Walnuts are super rich in omega-3s, and you should eat a dozen or so every day. If taken regularly, walnuts can improve your brain health, balance cholesterol, maintain healthy blood pressure, and lower your risk of depression.

If you prefer almonds, having just a few of this protein- and vitamin E-rich nuts, you can easily reduce your cholesterol levels, improve insulin sensitivity, boost memory, and even be protected against breast cancer.

14. Green tea

Dr. Sebi

This is probably the healthiest tea there is. It's hard to believe that all you have to do to reap some of its many benefits, is take 2-3 cups a day. Green tea improves metabolism and helps with weight loss. It's rich in antioxidants and helps reduce the risk of certain types of cancer (eg breast, prostate, and colorectal). It is a mild stimulant and can improve your brain function. It lowers the risk of Alzheimer's and Parkinson's. It successfully kills oral bacteria and improves dental health. It lowers risk of type 2 diabetes and cardiovascular disease.

A recent study in Japan showed that those who drink 5 cups or more a day are least likely to die in the next 11 years.

15.   Turmeric

Indian cuisine cannot be imagined without this spice but it is only recently that we found out how healthy it is. Turmeric can help reduce arthritic pain, stop the growth of cancer cells, treat inflammatory skin conditions such as psoriasis and eczema, boost your immune system, improve brain function, support your heart, help you maintain healthy joints and bones, stimulate digestion, and even boost the production of serotonin and dopamine hormones that make you feel good.

Kat Marie-Claire

Chapter 6

Can Disease be Slowed Down or Reversed with a Diet?

Many conditions can be prevented or reversed with a diet. Actually, there are so many of those, that most of the diseases of modern times are known to be diet-related. One of the reasons so many new diets have been created over the last thirty years is that thanks to scientific advancements, we finally understand just how important nutrition is for both physical and mental health.

However, the science of nutrition does not only focus on diseases that can be prevented or reduced with a balanced diet. It also looks at how a poor diet and food intolerances contribute to certain conditions.

Managing Your Condition with a Diet

Education is the key to good health. Due to an alarming increase in life-threatening diseases, most of which are diet-related and therefore preventable, governments have intensified the promotion of healthy lifestyle habits both at home and at the workplace.

We know that our body requires certain nutrients for optimal health. Although there are nutrients that don't provide energy, i.e. water, they are still necessary for our body to function well. Some provide the bulk of our diet, i.e. macronutrients, while others are needed in very small quantities but are nevertheless essential for one's health, i.e. micronutrients.

Raising your awareness of the importance of a healthy diet is the first step in managing your health with a diet. If your current eating habits are less than good, being aware of what you stand to gain if you adopt a balanced diet, can serve as a powerful motivation.

Kat Marie-Claire

Benefits of A Healthy Diet
1. You reduce the risk of some diseases
2. You maintain a healthy blood pressure
3. You maintain healthy cholesterol levels
4. You strengthen your immune system
5. You have more energy
6. Your mood improves

A healthy diet is a source of energy as well as nutrients your body needs to function well. However, certain conditions or phases of your life may require a special diet.

For example, there is a difference between a healthy diet for weight loss, high blood sugar level, or diabetes. Similarly, a healthy diet for a professional athlete, a pregnant woman, or a person in their 70s, need to satisfy very specific individual requirements.

In other words, a healthy diet is not a one-size-fits-all. Rather, it is a dietary regimen that provides nutrition YOUR body needs to stay alive, healthy, lower its blood pressure, lose weight, etc. When your diet contains all the nutrients you need, it easily creates new cells or repairs the damaged ones. In other words, a nutritious diet enables the body to self-heal and self-repair.

An important thing to be taken into account when choosing a diet is knowing how your body responds to certain foods. For example, milk is a good source of calcium but if you are lactose intolerant, drinking milk or having a lot of dairy products in your diet will create more harm than good.

Besides, not all diets suit everyone. The choice of a diet becomes particularly important if you have a chronic condition or if you are trying to prevent or reduce certain diseases. Fortunately, many of the common chronic conditions can be avoided, controlled or even reversed with the right nutrition. For example:

– Fatty liver
– Heart disease
– Stroke
– High blood pressure
– Certain types of cancer
– Obesity
– Osteoporosis

Dr. Sebi

- Anemia
- Type 2 diabetes
- Depression and anxiety
- Dental disease
- Insomnia
- Celiac disease
- Irritable bowel syndrome
- Adrenal Fatigue Syndrome
- Alzheimer's

Prevention is always better (and easier) than cure which is why it's very important to know that some of these conditions, e.g. obesity, diabetes, and high blood pressure increase the risk of other serious conditions, e.g. dementia.

Kat Marie-Claire

Chapter 7

HEALTH CONDITIONS DR. SEBI DIET CAN HEAL

The alkaline diet is very healthy although it is quite restrictive which means it requires both discipline and a thought-through approach. However, Dr. Sebi therapy's "secret" is the herbal tonics and teas he insisted his clients used alongside the strict alkaline diet.

A healthy diet, any diet, boosts one's immune system and improves one's health so what is so special about Dr. Sebi diet?

Overall, Dr. Sebi passionately believed that people in Africa, Asia or Europe are not genetically predisposed to eat the same kind of food. We all evolved in regions where Mother Nature made sure that all the ingredients necessary to help us stay healthy, were available locally. Dr. Sebi compares the diets of the Inuit people with that of the sub-Saharan African people. Neither population could stay healthy for very long if they were forced to live on the diet they were not genetically programmed to survive on.

So, Dr. Sebi bases his therapy on the premise that we all know where we, or our ancestors, come from and that our diet should reflect our place of origin. The local climate, as well as your genetic makeup, can give a very clear indication of what sort of foods are best for your health.

Due to global trade, we now eat a much more varied diet than was possible thirty years ago. This may not be such a good idea. Even the ancient Indian medical healing system of Ayurveda insists the healthiest diet is the one based on local and seasonal foods.

Dr. Sebi claimed that his alkaline diet could help cure even untreatable diseases. His most famous treatments were for the following conditions:

Kat Marie-Claire

– **Herpes**

Herpes simplex virus is what causes cold sores most of us have experienced at some stage.

Cold sores are probably one of the most common types of herpes simplex. They appear in the corner of the mouth and are not only unsightly but also very painful, making it difficult to eat, brush your teeth or even open your mouth. Unfortunately the herpes virus is not curable, however, certain creams can quickly reduce both the pain and inflammation.

You are most likely to get cold sores if your immune system is weakened. So, the first line of defense is a strong immune system.

An inflammation you experience with herpes simplex infections is simply the way the body naturally heals itself. It is through an inflammatory process that the body gets rid of pathogens that are causing it harm. Cold sores and genital herpes can be very painful so to deal with this condition, you need something with anti-inflammatory and pain-relieving properties.

According to Dr. Sebi, curing herpes requires thorough body-cleansing and consumption of iron-containing products.

The goal is to create an environment where herpes cannot survive. To start with, your cells need oxygen to function well and using synthetic drugs to deal with your condition (regardless of what it is), you rob the cells of oxygen.

So, when curing herpes, Dr. Sebi pays particular attention to a diet.

While trying to get rid of herpes, you should stay away from starches, sweets, chickpeas, avocado, and quinoa. Instead, you should focus on bitter foods, such as lettuce, zucchini, squash, mushrooms, cactus plant flower or leaf, and sea vegetables.

Herbs known to help cure herpes that can be brewed as tea are burdock, dandelion, and yellow dock. Take 3 cups a day for at least ten days, or until the condition clears. You can have these teas individually, or you can mix equal quantities of these three herbs and store the mixture in a glass container.

Fasting also helps because it cleanses the body. The more rigorous the fast, the sooner will you get rid of your problem. If you start feeling weak, take a couple of dates. According to Dr. Sebi, all diseases boil down to one disease which occurs when the mucous membrane is damaged. The mucous membrane protects the cells and should not be compromised in any way. If it is, the cells it's been protecting become vulnerable to pathogens.

– Diabetes

Dr. Sebi alkaline diet, which is slightly different from the standard alkaline diet, successfully treats diabetes provided one strictly follows the Dr. Sebi dietary regimen and uses herbal tonics or teas known to be particularly beneficial for diabetes, eg fig leaf, mulberry leaf, and black seed.

– Impotence

According to Dr. Sebi, the cure is simple – fast until your erectile dysfunction is cleared. Drink plenty of alkaline water of pH 7 and above and take some of Dr. Sebi herbal supplements. What seems to boost the blood flow to the penis particularly well, is the burdock root juice.

– AIDS

Dr. Sebi believed that to cure AIDS, you start by cleansing the mucous membranes throughout the body, eg on the skin, in the blood, in the lymphatic system, etc. So, there is no special herbal supplement that treats AIDS. Instead, Dr. Sebi's treatment revolves around simultaneously cleansing various organs and systems and providing the body with an adequate diet, including some healing herbs.

Regardless of how well you think you eat, chances are your body is starved of "real food." It has probably, unbeknown to you, been slowly but steadily poisoned by a diet rich in sugar, starch, animal protein, and synthetic drugs. So, to fight off infection and disease, especially a disease like AIDS, your needs to be regenerated and rehydrated. And that is what the purpose of Dr. Sebi alkaline diet is.

– Alzheimer's

Dr. Sebi claimed that all diseases are caused by mucous, ie mucous in a particular organ or system causes the deterioration of that organ, eg sinusitis, bronchitis, pneumonia, etc.

So, if there is excess mucous in the brain, you become vulnerable to neurodegenerative disorders, eg Alzheimer's, Parkinson's, dementia, etc. To prevent the onset of disease (any disease), the body should be regularly cleansed of mucous.

The brain needs oxygen. When a lot of mucus has accumulated in the brain, it causes inflammation, which in turn prevents oxygen from flowing freely. So, treating all brain conditions starts with cleansing the brain of the accumulated mucuous.

The brain is the only organ that produces electricity. It does that through copper/carbon interaction.

Although most people enjoy acidic foods, eg dairy, meat, and starch, this diet is very stressful to the body. Our body needs iron because it helps with the transfer of oxygen to the brain. If your iron levels are low, the oxygen supply to the brain is slowed down. This is why Dr. Sebi recommends the so-called "electric foods", ie alkaline foods high in iron, as a treatment for all brain conditions.

Besides, for neurological disorders, Dr. Sebi insists on consuming alkaline water of pH7 and above and on foods rich in oxygen, eg avocados, watercress, apples, berries, dates, mango, and papaya.

In summary, reversing a condition with a diet is not only possible but is the only 100% natural and sustainable long-term solution. Depending on the seriousness of your disease, as well as your self-discipline, results may be achieved in as little as a few weeks or, in case of some conditions, a couple of years. Needless to say, it's much easier to prevent a disease than to cure it.

Dr. Sebi

CHAPTER 8

DIABETES

According to the World Health Organization (WHO), about 1.5 million people die from diabetes every year. However, when we know that 18 million people die annually from cardiovascular diseases caused by diabetes and hypertension, we can begin to understand just how big a problem this condition is.

The Diabetes Epidemic

Diabetes is a complex disease that medical science still does not fully understand. Globally, there's been a steady increase in noncommunicable diseases, or the so-called diseases of civilization, one of which is diabetes.

80% of all diabetics live in developing countries, and the disease is spreading particularly fast in populations that have undergone major lifestyle changes. This highlights the importance of lifestyle choices. Just like a lifestyle change can trigger the onset of diabetes, it can also reverse it.

There are two types of diabetes:

- **Type 1 diabetes**

Type 1 diabetes develops usually in children and young adults. It is an autoimmune disorder that happens when the immune system destroys its pancreatic beta cells. These are the cells that make insulin, a hormone that controls blood sugar. Those affected with this type of diabetes need to take regular insulin injections.

- **Type 2 diabetes**

Type 2 diabetes is the kind that affects adults, mainly those in the 40-60 age group. The disease starts as insulin resistance ie a condition when cells cannot use insulin properly so the pancreas eventually stops producing it. What's particularly worrying about this condition is that those affected by it are 2-4 times more likely to develop cardiovascular disease. Of those who do, 80% die from it.

There is also the prediabetes, a condition when the blood sugar level is higher than normal but still not high enough for someone to be diagnosed with type 2 diabetes.

Fortunately, this condition can be easily controlled and reversed with weight loss and physical activity. However, if unaddressed, about 30% of individuals diagnosed with prediabetes will develop full-blown type 2 diabetes within 5 years.

Fortunately, having prediabetes does not mean you will develop type 2 diabetes. The disease is easily preventable.

However, there is a conflict between alternative and mainstream medicine approach to diabetes. While alternative and integrative medicine call for a lifestyle change, conventional medicine and pharmaceutical companies advocate treating the disease with synthetic drugs.

If you are told you have prediabetes, it signifies that your blood sugar level is higher than normal, but still not high enough to cause alarm. However, without a major lifestyle change, you are very likely to develop type 2 diabetes. So, although prediabetes is not a disease as such it should be taken seriously because it means that deterioration of your heart, blood vessels, and kidney have already started.

Fortunately, all it takes to bring your blood sugar level back to normal is a change of diet and weight management.

Diabetes Risk Factors and Symptoms

Being overweight or obese is the main risk factor for type 2 diabetes simply because increased weight leads to insulin resistance. The good news is that this risk factor is easily avoided. Studies show that if you reduce your weight by as little as 5%, you can easily prevent the onset of 2 diabetes.

The main cause of diabetes is the mismatch between how we were genetically predisposed to live and how we end up living. Not only do we often make unhealthy food choices, we also eat much more than we actually need for maintenance. The surplus is stored sd fat deposits. Over the years, as our weight grows and our vitality steadily declines, our health takes a blow. Our mental health declines as our quality of life drops, we become vulnerable to heart disease, stroke, and some types of cancer. And of course, diabetes which, if not managed can lead to blindness, kidney failure, and heart disease.

Dr. Sebi

Main Causes of Diabetes

– **Obesity**

Today, there is a major imbalance between the amount of food we take and the energy we expend during the day. Most people living in urban areas lead sedentary lifestyles. Being overweight is bad enough but obesity is the root cause of many life-threatening diseases. Poor diet and a sedentary lifestyle can easily turn anyone from being overweight to being obese.

– **Genetics**

Unfortunately, we have no control over genes we inherit from our ancestors. However, if you know you have a family history of diabetes, you can easily avoid the onset of disease by introducing some lifestyle changes as soon as possible.

– **Longer life expectancy**

Type 2 diabetes usually affects middle-aged people. At the time when life expectancy was about 50, very few individuals lived long enough to develop this disease.

– **Processed foods**

Many blame processed foods for the alarming rise of type 2 diabetes. Food processing is known to produce certain chemicals, eg oxidized ascorbic acid and lipoic acid, which contribute to the development of diabetes. Even infant formula is high in these harmful ingredients.

While prediabetes usually comes with no particular symptoms, type 2 diabetes is preceded with certain tell-tale signs:

– Darkened skin on the neck, armpits, elbows, knees, and knuckles
– Increased thirst
– Frequent urination
– Fatigue
– Blurred vision

Although there is nothing you can do about your genetic makeup or age, there are relatively easy ways to prevent or even reverse this potentially very serious chronic condition.

Kat Marie-Claire

Chapter 9

REVERSING FULL-BLOWN DIABETES WITH A LIFESTYLE CHANGE

You may be unaware of it but education is key for better health. If you know what lifestyle changes you need to make to avoid certain diseases, and you choose not to make them, you have only yourself to blame for the consequences. Being well-informed, ie knowing what you are up against is half the battle. Most diseases come with certain symptoms that serve as a warning something is not right. The good thing about all diseases of civilization, including diabetes, is that they can be avoided, controlled or even reversed with a lifestyle change. And lifestyle is about personal habits and diet.

A sedentary lifestyle and poor diet are believed to be the two main causes of obesity. As obesity is the leading contributing factor for the development of type 2 diabetes, to avoid this condition, all you have to do is introduce these two changes into your lifestyle:

— **Physical activity**

The reason physical activity helps reduce the risk of diabetes is that it improves the way cells respond to insulin and lower blood sugar levels. Glucose is the main energy source for muscles, so the more muscle you have and the more physically active you are, the more glucose is removed from the blood. Besides, physical activity helps you maintain healthy weight.

— **Diabetes-friendly diet**

A diabetes diet is simply a diet based on nutrient-dense foods and low in fat and calories. It revolves around fruits, vegetables, and whole grains.

If you have full-blown diabetes or have been diagnosed with prediabetes, the best thing to do is consult a dietitian to help you create a personalized diet plan to control your blood sugar and manage weight.

Alternatively, you can follow the so-called "plate method." It's about eating more vegetables and fewer calories. For example;

Kat Marie-Claire

– ½ of your plate should be reserved for nonstarchy vegetables, eg spinach, carrots, tomatoes.
– ¼ of the plate should be reserved for protein, e.g. fish, lean meat or chicken
– ¼ of your place should be filled with whole-grains, eg brown rice, green peas, etc.
– You should also include some good fats, eg avocado or nuts.
– For dessert, you can have a piece of fruit or a piece of cheese

Chapter 10

HOW TO REVERSE DIABETES THE DR. SEBI WAY

Being diagnosed with diabetes means your blood sugar level is too high. It also means that your body either doesn't make insulin or doesn't use it as it should. Although potentially a dangerous condition, diabetes is not a death sentence.

An easy way of controlling or reversing this chronic condition is to keep your blood sugar level within the required range, have diabetes-friendly meals three times a day at regular times, and be physically active. These simple lifestyle changes will ensure your insulin is utilized better.

So, how do I start?

For diabetes, diet is key. Create a personalized meal plan by focusing on foods that support healthy insulin production and are rich in fiber, eg fruits, vegetables, legumes, and low-fat dairy.

- **Fiber-rich diet**

Fruits, vegetables, and legumes are the best natural source of fiber.

- **Healthy carbs**

Carbohydrates break down into glucose, so to control your blood sugar levels, learn how to calculate the amount of carbs you take in each meal or a snack. Healthy carbs are found in vegetables, fruit, legumes, potatoes, and whole grains.

- Glycemic index

Some people choose to use the glycemic index to select diabetes-friendly foods. This particularly applies to carbohydrates.

- **Omega 3-rich foods**

Omega-3 fatty acids not only have amazing health benefits, they also have the power to improve diabetes and reduce or prevent obesity. As obesity is a major risk factor for type 2 diabetes, all diabetics should eat salmon, mackerel, tuna, and sardines as often as possible.

– **Healthy fats**

These should be taken in moderation for although healthy, they are calorie-rich, eg avocado, nuts, and healthy oils (canola, olive, peanut).

– **Protein**

Diabetics can get protein from lean meats, poultry, fish, and dairy.

There are also foods that people with diabetes or prediabetes should stay away from:

– **Saturated fats**

These are found in high-fat dairy and animal products eg butter, beef, sausage and bacon, palm kernel oil.

– **Trans fats**

If you avoid processed foods, shortening, and stick margarine you will easily avoid this kind of fats.

– **Cholesterol**

Cholesterol is abundant in high-fat dairy products and high-fat animal proteins (eg fast foods, liver, bacon and fatty meats, high-fat dairy (eg butter, whipped cream), and egg yolks. Diabetics should avoid cholesterol or limit the intake to 200 mg per day.

– **Salt**

Eat as little salt as you can, but don't leave it out completely for this may cause other health problems. You should be particularly careful about salt if you have high blood pressure.

Most of the foods recommended for diabetes are the same as those recommended on Dr. Sebi alkaline diet. However, there are differences.

Similarities:
– Both diets are rich in fruits and vegetables
– Both diets recommend avoiding processed foods

Differences:
– Diabetes diet allows grains while Dr. Sebi alkaline diet forbids most grains
– Diabetes diet allows low-fat dairy products, while for an alkaline diet dairy is off-limits
– Alkaline diet doesn't allow most food-allergy triggers, eg milk, eggs, peanuts, walnuts, fish and shellfish while these foods are allowed on diabetes diet

Numerous studies show that many chronic diseases can be prevented with a plant-based diet, eg heart disease, cancer, autoimmune disorders, diabetes, muscular degeneration, etc.

Besides, laboratory studies suggest that introducing or withdrawing the animal protein intake can turn some diseases "on and off, like a switch."

In other words, animal-based foods increase the chance of disease, while nutrients from plant-based foods help the body repair itself.

However, the key thing to remember is that for a plant-based diet to work, one must use different parts of a plant, eg:

– Fruits (for vitamins)
– Leaves (for antioxidants and fiber)
– Roots (for complex carbs)
– Flowers (for antioxidants and phytochemicals)
– Fungi (for selenium and antioxidants)
– Whole grains (for healthy carbs)
– Legumes (for protein and fiber)

However, Dr. Sebi easily cured himself as well as many other people from diabetes by strictly following the alkaline diet which lacks many of the healthy foods recommended to diabetics. How did he do it?

Dr. Sebi-approved foods are the same as those approved on a general alkaline diet. This means that the alkaline diet excludes some of the foods which are recommended for diabetes-friendly diets, eg dairy, whole grains, eggs, certain nuts, etc.

However, what makes Dr. Sebi diet stand out is the use of healing herbs which supplement the standard alkaline diet.

The herbs can be used as tea, tonic, supplements, or added to dishes such as soups, smoothies, shakes, etc.

The Complete List of Dr. Sebi-Recommended Herbs

Bilberry - Berry and leaf
Bitter Melon - Fruit and seeds
Bladderwrack - Whole herb
Blueberry - Fruit and leaf

Burdock - Root
Dandelion - Root and leaf
Eucalyptus - Leaf
Fenugreek - Seeds
Fig - Fruit and leaf
Guaco - Root
Guinea Hen Weed {Anamu} - Whole plant
Ginger - Root
Huereque {Wereke} - Root
Holy Basil - Leaf
Irish Sea Moss - Whole herb
Linden {Tila} - Flower and leaf
Mango - Fruit and leaf
Milk Thistle -Seeds
Mulberry - Leaf
Nettle - Leaf
Nopal Cactus - Flat stems
Okra - Whole and seeds
Prickly Pear Cactus - Whole fruit, seeds, and juice
Prodigiosa - Leaf
Raspberry -Berry and leaf
Sage - Leaf
Seville {Sour Orange} - Fruit
Soursop - Fruit and juice

3 Herbs Dr. Sebi Particularly Recommended For Diabetes

— **Fig leaf**

Fig leaf tea is a well-known natural remedy for diabetes. Alternatively, you can take a fig leaf extract. Research carried out in 2009 confirmed that fig leaves easily stabilize blood sugar levels. You should use two teaspoons of leaves per cup of water. Or, you can boil two spoonfuls of leaves per liter of water.

— **Mulberry leaf**

Mulberry leaves have been traditionally used to treat diabetes and obesity in Korea and Japan. If you'd rather use the extract, don't take more than one gram in a little bit

Dr. Sebi

of water before meals.

- **Black seed (cumin seed)**

Black seed oil successfully controls blood sugar levels and is traditionally used for treating diabetes all over the Middle East. You can use it as a black seed oil that you can add to cereal or salads, or as a powder which you can make as tea or sprinkle over meals. Even as little as 2 teaspoons of black seed powder a day is enough to reverse diabetes.

Other plants recommended for diabetes for the Dr. Sebi treatment are bitter melon, avocado, Swiss chard, red clover, fenugreek, ginger, okra, and ginseng
In summary, adopting healthy living habits and a healthy eating plan is the easiest and the most natural way to address diabetes. Maintaining a healthy weight and following a plant-based diet will not only help you reverse this condition but will go a long way to ensuring you reduce the risk of many other chronic diseases.

Kat Marie-Claire

Chapter 11

DR. SEBI ALKALINE RECIPES

Breakfast

SPELT WAFFLE

Preparation Time: 10 Minutes | **Cooking Time**: 15 Minutes | **Servings**: 4
Ingredients:
- 1 cup Spelt Flour
- 1 tsp. Sea Moss
- ¼ cup Hemp Milk
- Pinch of Sea Salt
- ½ tsp. Allspice Powder

Method of Preparation:
1) To begin with, brush the waffle maker with the oil.
2) After that, preheat the waffle maker.
3) Next, pour the batter into the maker.
4) Cook the waffles for 5 to 6 minutes on medium heat or until browned.
5) Serve it warm.

BLUEBERRY CAKE

Preparation Time: 10 Minutes | **Cooking Time**: 45 Minutes | **Servings**: Makes 6 Muffins
Ingredients:
- 1 cup Chickpea Flour
- 1 cup Blueberries
- 2/3 cup + 1 tbsp. Spelt Flour
- Dash of Sea Salt
- ¾ cup Water
- 2 tbsp. Grapeseed Oil
- 6 tbsp. Agave Nectar

Method of Preparation:
1) To start with, place all the ingredients needed to make in a high-speed blender and blend for 3 minutes until they are no more lumps in it.
2) Next, transfer the mixture to a parchment paper-lined baking sheet and spread it across evenly.
3) After that, bake it for 28 to 30 minutes or until browned and cooked.

Banana Nut Muffins

Preparation Time: 10 Minutes | **Cooking Time**: 40 Minutes | **Servings**: Makes 12 to 14 slices

Ingredients:
- 3 ½ cup Spelt Flour ; ½ cup Agave Syrup
- 3 Bananas, mashed ; Spring Water, as needed
- 1 cup Walnuts, chopped; Pinch of Salt
- ¼ cup Date Syrup ; ¾ cup Perrier

Method of Preparation:
1) For making this delicious cake, combine the mashed banana, date syrup, and agave syrup in a large mixing bowl until mixed well.
2) Once combined, stir in the spelt flour and salt. Mix again.
3) Then, pour the Perrier along with the walnuts. Stir well.
4) If the batter seems too thickened, add more water as needed.
5) Now, pour the batter into the muffin molds and fill them 3/4th.
6) Finally, bake them at 350 ° F for 18 to 20 minutes or until cooked.

Teff Porridge

Preparation Time: 10 Minutes | **Cooking Time**: 10 Minutes | **Servings**: Makes 2

Ingredients:
- 2 cups Spring Water; 5 cups Teff Grain
- Dash of Sea Salt; 2 tbsp. Agave Syrup

Method of Preparation:
1) First, boil water in a pot over medium-high heat, and once it starts boiling, stir in the teff grains and salt.
2) Next, cover the lid of the pot and reduce the heat.
3) Now, allow it to simmer for 10 to 15 minutes or until cooked.
4) Garnish with more blueberries and agave syrup if desired.

Quinoa Porridge with Apple

Preparation Time: 10 Minutes | **Cooking Time**: 10 Minutes | **Servings**: 4

Ingredients:
- ½ of 1 Key Lime
- 5 cup Quinoa; 1 Apple, grated
- 1 tbsp. Coconut Oil; 1-inch Ginger

Method of Preparation:
1) To start with, cook the quinoa by following the instructions given in the packet.
2) Five minutes before the cooking time, add the grated apple.
3) Now, cook for half a minute and then spoon in lemon zest and lemon juice to it.
4) Next, pour the coconut oil into it and mix it well.
5) Finally, distribute the mixture among the serving bowls and garnish it with the ginger grated.

Dr. Sebi

Vegetable Omelet

Preparation Time: 10 Minutes | **Cooking Time**: 10 Minutes | **Servings**: Makes 1 Omelet
Ingredients:
- ¼ tsp. Oregano
- ¼ cup Garbanzo Beans Flour
- ¼ cup Mushrooms, chopped
- ¼ cup Roma Tomato, chopped
- ¼ cup Green Pepper, diced
- ¼ cup Onion, chopped
- ¼ tsp. Pure Sea Salt
- 1 tbsp. Grapeseed Oil
- ¼ tsp. Onion Powder
- 1/3 cup Spring Water
- ¼ tsp. Basil, sweet
- ¼ tsp. Cayenne Powder

Method of Preparation:
1) Begin by placing the garbanzo bean flour, water, and seasoning to a large mixing bowl. Whisk the mixture well until everything is well incorporated.
2) After that, heat the oil in a large skillet over medium-high heat.
3) Once the oil becomes hot, stir in a spoonful of all the veggies along with tomato.
4) Saute them for 2 to 3 minutes or until they become slightly tender.
5) Now pour the flour mixture to it and mix well.
6) Allow the mixture to cook for 4 minutes and then turn them over.
7) With a spatula, lift the sides of the omelet and tilt it slightly to the raised area so that all portions get cooked. Serve them hot.

Herbal Bread

Preparation Time: 10 Minutes | **Cooking Time**: 10 Minutes | **Servings**: Makes 1 loaf
Ingredients:
- 1 tbsp. Onion Powder
- 1 tsp. Oregano
- 1 tsp. Basil
- 1 tsp. Thyme
- ½ cup Date Syrup
- 1 ½ cup Spring Water
- 3 tbsp. Grapeseed Oil
- 4 cups Chickpeas Flour
- 1 tbsp. Pure Sea Salt

Method of Preparation:
1) Start by stirring all the dry ingredients in a medium-sized bowl until combined well.
2) After that, pour 1 cup of the spring water, date syrup, and grapeseed oil to it.

3) Mix well until you get a smooth batter. If the mixture seems too thick, add more water.
4) Now, pour the batter to the greased loaf pan and top it with herbs of your choice.
5) Finally, heat the oven to 350 °F and bake for 50 to 60 minutes.
6) Allow it to cool and serve.

SPELT GRANOLA

Preparation Time: 5 Minutes | **Cooking Time**: 10 Minutes | **Servings**: 4 to 6
Ingredients:
- ½ tsp. Pure Sea Salt
- ¼ cup Hemp Seeds
- ¼ cup Pumpkin Seeds
- 2 tbsp. Avocado Oil
- ½ cup Walnuts, chopped
- 2 cups Spelt Flakes

Method of Preparation:
1) To begin with, preheat the oven to 300 °F.
2) Next, place all the ingredients needed to make the granola in a large mixing bowl.
3) Combine well until you get a sticky mixture.
4) Now, transfer the mixture to a greased parchment paper-lined baking sheet and spread it out evenly.
5) Finally, bake for 8 minutes or until they are toasted.

KAMUT PORRIDGE

Preparation Time: 5 Minutes
Cooking Time: 15 Minutes
Servings: 2
Ingredients:
- 1 cup Kamut
- 2 cups Spring Water
- ¼ tsp. Cayenne Pepper
- ¼ tsp. Oregano
- ½ tsp. Pure Sea Salt
- ½ tsp. Pure Sea Salt

Method of Preparation:
1) To begin with, place 2 cups of the water in a medium-sized bowl.
2) After that, blend the Kamut to the saucepan and bring the mixture to a boil.
3) If the porridge is thickened, add more water.
4) Serve and enjoy.

BLUEBERRY SPELT PANCAKES

Preparation Time: 5 Minutes
Cooking Time: 15 Minutes
Servings: 2
Ingredients:
- 2 cups Spelt Flour
- ¼ tsp. Sea Moss
- 1 cup Hemp Milk
- ½ cup Agave Syrup
- ½ cup Spring Water
- ½ cup Blueberries
- 2 tbsp. Grapeseed Oil

Method of Preparation:
1) For making this healthy breakfast dish, combine spelt flour, grape seed oil, agave syrup, and sea moss in a large mixing bowl.
2) Now, pour the hemp milk and water to it gradually.
3) Then, fold in the blueberries into it gently.
4) After that, heat a large skillet over medium-high heat.
5) Once the skillet becomes hot, brush it with oil.
6) Next, spoon a ladle of the batter to it and cook for 3 to 5 minutes per side.
7) Serve them hot.

APPLE QUINOA PORRIDGE

Preparation Time: 5 Minutes
Cooking Time: 15 Minutes
Servings: 3 to 4
Ingredients:
- 2 Apples
- 1 cup Coconut Milk
- ½ cup Quinoa
- 1 cup Spring Water
- 1 tbsp. Date Sugar
- 1 tbsp. Date Syrup

Method of Preparation:
1) First, cook the quinoa along with all the ingredients excluding apple in a medium-sized pot for 8 minutes or until the quinoa is cooked.
2) Once cooked, stir in the chopped apples.
3) Serve them hot.

Kamut Puffs

Preparation Time: 5 Minutes
Cooking Time: 15 Minutes
Servings: 2 to 3
Ingredients:
- 2 tbsp. Grapeseed Oil
- 2 tbsp. Agave Syrup
- ½ cup Kamut Flakes

Method of Preparation:
1) To start with, place the flakes along with oil and syrup in a medium-sized bowl and coat the flakes well with the coating.
2) After that, transfer the flakes to a parchment paper-lined baking sheet evenly in a single layer.
3) Serve warm.

Basics

CHEESE

Preparation Time: 5 Minutes | **Cooking Time**: 15 Minutes | **Servings**: Makes 1 cup
Ingredients:
- 1 cup Brazil Nuts, soaked
- ¼ tsp. Pure Sea Salt
- 1 tsp. Sea Moss Gel
- ½ cup Spring Water
- ½ tsp. Basil
- 1 tsp. Key Lime Juice
- ½ tsp. Oregano
- ¼ cup Hemp Seed Milk
- ½ tsp. Onion Powder

Method of Preparation:
1) For making this tasty cheese recipe, place all the ingredients needed to make the cheese in a high-speed blender.
2) Blend for 2 minutes for a rich, creamy paste.

HEMP MILK

Preparation Time: 5 Minutes | **Cooking Time**: 5 Minutes | **Servings**: 1 to 2
Ingredients:
- 1 cup Hemp Seeds, hulled
- 6 cup Spring Water

Method of Preparation:
1) To start with, place hemp seeds and water in a high-speed blender and blend them until they are smooth.
2) Next, pour the remaining water to the blender and blend again.
3) Finally, pass the mixture through a strainer and transfer to a serving glass.

WALNUT MILK

Preparation Time: 5 Minutes | Cooking Time: 5 Minutes | Servings: 1 to 2
Ingredients:
- 1 cup Walnuts, soaked for 5 to 6 hours
- ¼ tsp. Sea Salt
- 2 cups Spring Water
- 1 tbsp. Agave

Method of Preparation:
1) To begin with, place all the ingredients needed to make the milk in a high-speed blender. Blend them for 2 to 3 minutes or until smooth.
2) Pass the milk mixture through a strainer or cheesecloth. Serve and enjoy.

Tahini Paste

Preparation Time: 5 Minutes | Cooking Time: 5 Minutes | Servings: 1 to 2
Ingredients:
- 2 tsp. Grapeseed Oil
- 1 cup Sesame Seeds

Method of Preparation:
1) For making this paste, place the sesame seeds in the food processor and process them until you get a chunky powder.
2) Next, pour the oil to it and blend it until you get a buttery

Pizza Crust

Preparation Time: 5 Minutes | Cooking Time: 60 Minutes | Servings: 4
Ingredients:
- 1 cup Spring Water
- 1 ½ cup Spelt Flour
- ½ tsp. Onion Powder
- ½ tsp. Pure Sea Salt
- ½ tsp. Oregano
- ½ tsp. Salt

Method of Preparation:
1) First, preheat the oven to 350 ° F.
2) After that, combine all the ingredients, excluding water needed to make the crust in a large mixing bowl.
3) Once combined, pour ½ cup of water to the mixture and make a dough out of it. If needed, add more water.
4) Now, place the dough on the floored working station and roll it out with a rolling pin.
5) Then, place the dough onto a greased parchment paper-lined baking sheet and spread it across evenly on all sides.
6) Apply grape seed oil over it and then makes holes on it with the aid of a fork.
7) Finally, bake for 13 to 15 minutes or until cooked and slightly browned.

Cucumber Pickle

Preparation Time: 5 Minutes | Cooking Time: 20 Minutes
Servings: 4 to 6
Ingredients:
- 1 tbsp. Dill
- 1 cup Cucumber, sliced
- ½ tsp. Red Pepper, crushed
- ½ cup Spring Water
- 1 tsp. Coriander
- 1 tsp. Sea Salt

Dr. Sebi

- 1 tbsp. Key Lime Juice

Method of Preparation:
1) For making this tasty pickle, make slices out of the cucumber.
2) After that, crush the spices and then spoon it over the cucumber slices in a medium-sized bowl.
3) Now, stir in the remaining ingredients and give everything a good toss.
4) Serve after storing for a minimum of 2 hours and for a maximum of 6 to 8 hours.

AQUAFABA

Preparation Time: 5 Minutes | Cooking Time: 150 Minutes **| Servings**: Makes 2 cups
Ingredients:
- 6 cups Spring Water + for soaking
- 14 oz. Garbanzo Beans
- 1 tsp. Pure Sea Salt

Method of Preparation:
1) First, keep all the ingredients in a large pot along with water and salt.
2) Now, bring the mixture to a rolling boil.
3) Next, take the pot from heat and set it aside for half an hour.
4) Then, drain the water and then add water to it again.
5) Once water is added, heat the pot again over medium heat and cook for another 1 ½ hours.
6) Drain the water from the beans in a container. This drained water is aquafaba.
7) Store in the refrigerator until it needs to be used.

SPICY OIL

Preparation Time: 5 Minutes | Cooking Time: 10 Minutes + Infusion Time **| Servings:** Makes 1 cup
Ingredients:
- ¾ cup Grape Seed Oil
- 1 tbsp. Cayenne Pepper, crushed

Method of Preparation:
1) To begin with, place the oil and the pepper in a glass container.
2) Now, shake the mixture and allow it to infuse for a day.

WHIPPED CREAM

Preparation Time: 5 Minutes | Cooking Time: 10 Minutes **| Servings**: Makes 1 cup
Ingredients:
- 1 cup Aquafaba
- ¼ cup Agave Syrup

Method of Preparation:
1) First, mix the agave syrup and aquafaba in a medium-sized bowl.

2) Whisk the mixture with a hand mixer for 10 to 15 minutes or until you get a smooth cream.

Blackberry Jam

Preparation Time: 5 Minutes | Cooking Time: 10 Minutes **| Servings**: Makes 1 cup

Ingredients:
- ¾ cup Blackberries
- ¼ cup Sea Moss Gel
- 1 tbsp. Key Lime Juice
- 3 tbsp. Agave Syrup

Method of Preparation:
1) Start by placing the blackberries in a medium-sized pot over medium-high heat.
2) Continue stirring the mixture until you get a liquid mixture.
3) Once the berries have become tender, blend them in the blender until it becomes a smooth mixture without any lumps.
4) Now, return the mixture back to the pot.
5) Then, stir in the sea moss gel, agave syrup, and lime juice to the mixture.
6) Next, bring the mixture to a boil until it becomes thickened. Stir continuously.
7) Take the pot from the heat and allow it to cool. Serve and enjoy.

Ginger Tea

Preparation Time: 5 Minutes | Cooking Time: 10 Minutes **| Servings**: Makes 1 cup

Ingredients:
- 4 cups Spring Water
- 1 pinch of Cayenne
- 2-inch Ginger Root, chopped
- 2 tbsp. Key Lime Juice
- 2 sprigs of Dill
- 1 tsp. Agave Syrup

Method of Preparation:
1) To start with, bring the water to a boil in a large pot over medium-high heat.
2) After that, stir in the ginger root and dill to it.
3) Now, boil the tea for a further 5 minutes.
4) Next, transfer the tea to a large container.
5) Then, add lime juice to it and mix well.
6) Finally, spoon in cayenne and raw agave to the tea. Serve well.

Dr. Sebi

Lunch

WATERCRESS SALAD

Preparation Time: 5 Minutes | Cooking Time: 10 Minutes | Servings: 2
Ingredients:
- 1/8 tsp. Pure Sea Salt
- 4 cups Watercress, torn
- 2 tbsp. Olive Oil
- 1 Avocado, pitted, halved and sliced
- 2 tsp. Agave Syrup
- Cayenne Powder, as needed
- 2 Red Onions, sliced thinly
- 1 Seville Orange, peeled & cubed
- 2 tbsp. Key Lime Juice

Method of Preparation:
1) First, place the orange, onion, avocado, and watercress in a large mixing bowl.
2) After that, mix olive oil, agave syrup, cayenne powder, key lime juice, and sea salt in another bowl until combined well.
3) Now, spoon this olive oil dressing over the salad and toss well.
4) Serve the healthy salad and enjoy it thoroughly.

WILD RICE & MUSHROOMS

Preparation Time: 5 Minutes | Cooking Time: 8 Minutes | Servings: 3
Ingredients:
- 1 cup Mushrooms, chopped finely
- 1 tsp. Olive Oil
- 1 tsp. Sea Salt
- 1 cup Wild Rice, cooked
- ½ cup Kale

Method of Preparation:
1) To begin with, cook the kale along with a bit of oil in a medium-sized skillet over medium-high heat.
2) Now, cook them for 2 to 3 minutes or until they have wilted slightly. Transfer to a plate and keep it aside. Reserve the oil in it.
3) Then, stir in the mushrooms to the skillet and cook for 3 to 5 minutes.
4) Once browned, move the mushrooms to a plate.
5) Next, season the mushrooms with salt and pepper. Serve it along with the wild rice and kale.

Zucchini Quinoa Salad

Preparation Time: 10 Minutes | **Cooking Time:** 40 Minutes | **Servings:** Makes 12 to 14 slices

Ingredients:
- 1 tsp. Oregano
- 2 Spring Onion, finely chopped
- 3 tbsp. Olive Oil
- 2 Zucchini, large & sliced
- 2 tbsp. Grapeseed Oil
- Juice of 1 Key Lime
- 15 oz. can of Chickpeas
- 1 tsp. Onion Powder
- 5 cup Quinoa, cooked

Method of Preparation:
1) To begin with, spoon in one tablespoon of oil to a large skillet over medium heat.
2) After that, stir in the zucchini slices and cook them for 3 to 4 minutes or until tender. Next, spoon in the oregano and the remaining oil to the skillet.
3) Finally, add all the remaining ingredients to a large bowl along with the cooked zucchini. Toss well.

Kamut Patties

Preparation Time: 5 Minutes | **Cooking Time:** 30 Minutes | **Servings:** 4

Ingredients:
- ½ tsp. Cayenne Powder
- 3 cups Kamut Cereal, cooked
- 1 tbsp. Onion Powder
- 1 cup Red Onions, minced
- 2 tbsp. Grapeseed Oil
- 1 cup Spelt Flour
- 1 tbsp. Oregano
- 1 cup of Yellow & Green Bell Pepper, chopped
- 1 tbsp. Basil
- ½ cup Hempseed Milk
- Pure Sea Salt, as needed

Method of Preparation:
1) To begin with, combine Kamut cereal, hempseed oil, seasoning, and veggies in a large mixing bowl.
2) Next, spoon in ½ of the spelt flour into it and mix well until you get a dough.
3) Then, make patties out of this dough.
4) After that, spoon in grapeseed oil into a heated large skillet over medium-high heat. Once the oil becomes hot, place the patties on the pan.
5) Now, cook the patties for 5 to 6 minutes or until golden brown.
6) Serve them hot.

Dr. Sebi

KALE SALAD

Preparation Time: 5 Minutes | **Cooking Time**: 5 Minutes | **Servings**: 1
Ingredients:
- 1 Avocado, diced
- Dash of Cayenne Pepper
- Juice of 1 Lime
- 1 Cucumber, small
- 6 to 8 Cherry Tomatoes
- ½ of 1 Purple Onion, sliced
- Sea Salt, as needed
- 1 tbsp. Grapeseed Oil

Method of Preparation:
1) To start with, place all the ingredients in a large mixing bowl and toss them until everything is well incorporated. Serve and enjoy.

MUSHROOM SOUP

Preparation Time: 5 Minutes | **Cooking Time**: 45 Minutes | **Servings**: 6
Ingredients:
- 2 tbsp. Grapeseed Oil
- 3 cups Mushrooms, sliced
- 1 tsp. Cayenne Powder
- 1 ½ cup Garbanzo Beans Flour
- 2 tsp. Basil, torn
- 1 cup Onion, mashed
- 2 tsp. Pure Sea Salt
- 2 cups Chayote Squash, peeled & cubed
- 1 tbsp. Onion Powder
- 1 cup Hempseed Milk
- 1 tsp. Cayenne Pepper
- 1 cup Aquafaba

Method of Preparation:
1) Begin by spooning oil to a large pot and heat it over medium heat.
2) Once the oil becomes slightly hot, stir in the onion and mushrooms.
3) Cook them for 5 minutes or until transparent and tender.
4) Next, spoon in the hempseed milk, aquafaba, and four cups of spring water to the pot. Then, stir in the squash cubes along with the seasonings. Mix well.
5) Now, bring the mixture to a boil.
6) In the meantime, blend the garbanzo bean flour and the remaining spring water in the blender for 1 to 1 ½ minutes or until it is smooth without any lumps.
7) Finally, pour the flour mixture to the pot and give everything a good stir.
8) Cook the mixture for 30 minutes or until thickened while stirring it occasionally.
9) Serve it hot and enjoy it.

Chickpeas Salad

Preparation Time: 5 Minutes
Cooking Time: 5 Minutes
Servings: 3
Ingredients:

- 1 ½ cups Chickpeas, drained & rinsed
- ½ cup Red Onion, diced
- ¼ cup Cilantro, fresh & chopped
- 1 cup Avocado
- Sea Salt, to taste

Method of Preparation:
1) To begin with, place chickpeas in a large bowl and mash it with a masher.
2) Then, mash the avocado and combine it well.
3) After that, pour lemon juice into the mixture and mix it well.
4) Next, stir in the cilantro and lime juice. Stir again.
5) Now, spoon in salt. Stir again.
6) Serve and enjoy.

Cucumber Mushroom Salad

Preparation Time: 5 Minutes
Cooking Time: 10 Minutes
Servings: 2
Ingredients:

- 1 tsp. Olive Oil
- 5 Mushrooms, halved
- Juice from ½ of 1 Key Lime
- 10 Olives
- 6 Cherry Tomatoes, halved
- Pure Sea Salt, as needed
- 6 Lettuce leaves washed
- ½ of 1 Cucumber, chopped

Method of Preparation:
1) For making this easy healthy salad, place the lettuce leaves, tomatoes, mushrooms, olives, and cucumber in a large mixing bowl.
2) To this, spoon in the olive oil and key lime juice over the salad. Toss well.
3) Next, sprinkle the sea salt over it.
4) Toss well and enjoy it.

Tacos

Preparation Time: 5 Minutes | Cooking Time: 15 Minutes | Servings: 2 to 3

Ingredients:
- 1 cup Garbanzo Beans, cooked
- 2 Plum Tomatoes, chopped
- 2 Avocadoes, mashed
- ½ of 1 Key Lime
- 1 Onion, small & chopped
- Sea Salt, as needed
- 1 Bell Pepper, chopped
- Spelt Flour Tortillas, as needed
- Cilantro, as needed

Method of Preparation:
1) First, combine the mashed avocadoes with tomatoes, onion, and bell pepper in a medium bowl.
2) After that, season it with sea salt.
3) Then, heat the garbanzo beans and the spelt flour tortillas.
4) Fill it with mashed guacamole and garnish with cilantro.

Macaroni & Cheese

Preparation Time: 5 Minutes | Cooking Time: 40 Minutes | Servings: 10

Ingredients:
- 2 tsp. Grapeseed Oil
- 12 oz. Alkaline Pasta
- Juice from ½ of 1 Key Lime
- 2 tsp. Onion Powder
- ¼ cup Garbanzo Flour
- 1 tsp. Pure Sea Salt
- 1 cup Spring Water
- 1 cup Brazil Nuts, raw & soaked for overnight
- 1 cup Hempseed Milk
- ½ tsp. Achiote, grounded

Method of Preparation:
1) To begin with, cook the pasta by following the instructions given on the packet until al dente.
2) Next, preheat the oven to 350° F.
3) Then, transfer the cooked pasta to a baking pan and drizzle oil over it.
4) Now, place all the remaining ingredients in a high-speed blender and blend for 2 minutes or until you get a smooth sauce.
5) After that, pour the sauce over the cooked pasta and toss well.
6) Finally, bake the pasta for 28 to 30 minutes.
7) Serve and enjoy.

Quinoa Rice

Preparation Time: 5 Minutes | Cooking Time: 50 Minutes | Servings: 2

Ingredients:
- ¼ of 1 Onion, diced
- 1 cup Quinoa, cooked
- ½ of 1 Bell Pepper, cubed
- ½ tbsp. Grapeseed Oil
- ½ cup Zucchini, cubed
- ½ tsp. Pure Sea Salt
- ½ cup Mushroom, sliced
- ¼ tsp. Cayenne Pepper or as needed

Method of Preparation:
1) For making this tasty rice fare, spoon in the oil to a heated medium-sized saucepan over medium heat.
2) Once the oil becomes hot, stir in the onion and cook them for 4 minutes or until slightly browned.
3) Then, spoon in the mushrooms, bell peppers, and zucchini to it and continue cooking for further 4 minutes or until the veggies are tender.
4) Now, stir in the cooked quinoa to the saucepan and mix well until everything is well incorporated. Cook until the rice becomes slightly browned.
5) Finally, transfer them to a serving bowl and serve it hot.

Amaranth with Pears

Preparation Time: 5 Minutes | Cooking Time: 10 Minutes | Servings: 4

Ingredients:
- ½ cup Walnuts, chopped & Currants
- 1 cup Amaranth
- Pinch of Salt
- 3 cups Spring Water
- 1 tbsp. Agave Syrup
- ½ of 1 Pear
- 1 tbsp. Coconut Oil

Method of Preparation:
1) Begin by placing water in a medium-sized saucepan.
2) Boil the mixture, and once it begins to boil, stir in the amaranth.
3) Now, allow it to simmer for 9 to 12 minutes or until cooked while stirring it occasionally. Once the mixture starts thickening and has a creamy consistency, take the pan from the stove.
4) Next, spoon in all the remaining ingredients to another saucepan and give a good stir. Cook on medium heat for 2 to 3 minutes.
5) Finally, add the mixture to the cooked amaranth and mix well.
6) Serve warm.

Garbanzo Bean Burger

Preparation Time: 5 Minutes | Cooking Time: 40 Minutes **| Servings**: 4
Ingredients:
- ½ tsp. Cayenne Pepper
- 1 cup Garbanzo Flour
- 2 tsp. Pure Sea Salt
- ½ cup Kale, diced
- ½ tsp. Cayenne Powder
- 1 Plum Tomato, diced
- 1 tsp. Dill
- ½ cup Green Peppers, diced
- 2 tsp. Oregano
- ½ cup Onion, diced
- ½ cup Spring Water
- 2 tsp. Basil
- 2 tbsp. Grapeseed Oil
- 2 tsp. Onion Powder

For the burger:
- 8 Flatbreads
- 1 cup Sauce
- 2 Plum Tomatoes, sliced
- 1 Red Onion, sliced

Method of Preparation:
1) First, mix all the spices and vegetables to a large mixing bowl and then spoon in the garbanzo flour to it.
2) To this, pour the spring water gradually. Combine everything until you get a dough. Tip: If it seems too loose, add more flour.
3) Now make cutlets out of this dough.
4) Next, heat the oil in a medium-sized skillet over medium-high heat.
5) Once the oil becomes hot, lower the heat to medium and then add the cutlets to it.
6) Cook the cutlets for 4 minutes or until golden browned in color.
7) After that, take a flatbread and keep the burger in it along with the onion, tomato, and sauce. Serve and enjoy it.

Gazpacho Soup

Preparation Time: 5 Minutes | Cooking Time: 15 Minutes **| Servings**: 2
Ingredients:
- 2 cups Spring Water
- 2 Basil Leaves
- 1 Avocado, ripe
- Juice from 1 Lime
- 1 Cucumber, peeled & seeds discarded

- ¼ tsp. Pure Sea Salt

Method of Preparation:
1) To start with, place all the ingredients, excluding the sea salt in the refrigerator.
2) After that, transfer the ingredients to a high-speed blender and blend them for 1 to 2 minutes or until you get a smooth soup with a bit of chunk.
3) Next, pour the soup to a container and keep it in the refrigerator until served.
4) Before serving, season it with salt and garnish it with the basil leaves. Tip: If you prefer, you can top it with thinly sliced cucumbers.
5) Serve and enjoy it.

Spaghetti Squash

Preparation Time: 5 Minutes | Cooking Time: 15 Minutes | Servings: 4

Ingredients:
- 1 Squash
- ¼ tsp. Onion Powder
- 1 tsp. Grapeseed Oil
- Pure Sea Salt, as needed
- ¼ tsp. Cayenne Pepper

Method of Preparation:
1) Preheat the oven to 325 ° F.
2) Next, slice the squash into halves and remove the seeds.
3) Then, brush the squash with oil and season it with the seasoning as need.
4) Now, place the squash on a greased baking sheet with the cut side down.
5) Bake for 38 minutes or until the squash is tender. Allow it to cool for 5 minutes.
6) Finally, run down the squash with a fork to get spaghetti strands.
7) Serve with butter and pepper if desired.

Dr. Sebi

Snacks

AMARANTH CRACKERS

Preparation Time: 10 Minutes | **Cooking Time**: 5 Minutes | **Servings**: 2
Ingredients:
- ½ cup Amaranth Flour, whole
- 1 tsp. Olive Oil
- 1 ½ cup Spring Water
- Sea Salt, to taste

Method of Preparation:
1) To start with, boil water in a deep saucepan over medium-high heat.
2) Next, stir in the amaranth and cook them for 25 to 30 minutes or until thickened, which has a consistency similar to thick oatmeal. Allow the mixture to cool and then place it in the refrigerator until chilled.
3) Preheat the oven to 425 ° F. Then, line a pizza pan with parchment paper and brush it with olive oil. Now, with a spoon, scoop the batter and make a circle on the parchment paper.
4) Apply it with olive oil and sprinkle salt over it.
5) Finally, bake for 20 minutes or until the bottom of the crust dries out and edges get crisper.
6) Remove the parchment paper and bake more if you want it crisper.

ONION RINGS

Preparation Time: 10 Minutes | **Cooking Time**: 30 Minutes | **Servings**: 8
Ingredients:
- ½ cup Aquafaba
- 3 tbsp. Grapeseed Oil
- 2 tsp. Pure Sea Salt
- 4 Sweet Onions
- 2 tsp. Oregano; 1 tsp. Cayenne Powder
- ½ cup Hempseed Milk
- 2 tsp. Onion Powder
- 1 cup Spelt Flour

Method of Preparation:
1) For making this delicious snack fares, preheat the oven to 450 ° F.
2) Next, combine the hempseed milk and Aquafiba in another medium bowl.
3) To this, add one teaspoon of oregano, sea salt and onion powder along with a half teaspoon of cayenne powder. Mix well.
4) After that, slice the onions about 1/4th inch into rings.
5) Now, place the spelt flour, remaining oregano, onion powder, sea salt, and cayenne powder in a container. Shake well.
6) Then, dip the onion first in the wet mixture and later in the spelt flour mixture.
7) Finally, arrange the onion slices on the greased baking sheet and brush them with oil.
8) Bake them for 10 to 15 minutes or until golden brown colored. Cool before serving.

Chickpea French Fries

Preparation Time: 10 Minutes | **Cooking Time**: 1 Hour 40 Minutes | **Servings**: 8

Ingredients:
- 1 tsp. Sea Salt
- ½ cup Onion, minced
- 2 cups Chickpea Flour
- 1 tsp. Cayenne
- 1 tbsp. Oregano
- ½ cup Green Bell Peppers, diced
- 2 tbsp. Grapeseed Oil
- 4 cups Spring Water
- 1 tbsp. Onion Powder

Method of Preparation:
1) For making this lip-smacking fare, you need to boil the water in a large pot over medium heat. Reduce the heat and stir in the chickpea flour to it gradually.
2) Then add the onions, seasonings, and bell pepper to it.
3) Cook the chickpea mixture for 10 minutes or until thickened while stirring it occasionally.
4) Now, pour the mixture to a parchment paper-lined baking sheet greased with the oil.
5) Spread the mixture evenly with a spatula and keep another parchment paper on top.
6) Next, place the sheet in the freezer for 20 minutes.
7) When the time is up, cut them in any shape preferred.
8) After that, preheat the oven to 400 ° F or 200 °C.
9) Finally, take another parchment paper-lined baking sheet which is greased with oil and keep the pieces in it.
10) Bake them for 20 minutes. Then flip them over. Continue cooking for further 10 minutes or until golden brown.
11) Serve them hot and enjoy it.

Chickpea Patties

Preparation Time: 5 Minutes | **Cooking Time**: 25 Minutes | **Servings**: 3 to 4

Ingredients:
- 1 tsp. Pure Sea Salt
- 2 cups Spring Water
- 1 tsp. Parsley
- 1 cup Garbanzo Flour

Method of Preparation
1) Begin by combining the garbanzo flour with the parsley, sea salt, and parsley in a large mixing bowl with a whisker until mixed well.
2) Now pour the mixture to a greased baking sheet and spread it across evenly.
3) Then, bake at 350 ° F or until golden brown colored.
4) Serve and enjoy.

BAKED NUTS

Preparation Time: 10 Minutes | **Cooking Time**: 10 Minutes | **Servings**: 4
Ingredients:
- ½ cup Hemp Seeds
- 1 cup Walnuts; 1 tsp. Olive Oil
- 1 cup Brazil Nuts; 1 tsp. Sesame Seeds

Method of Preparation:
1) First, preheat the oven to 350 ° F.
2) Next, toss all the nuts and hemp seeds in a mixing bowl until combined well.
3) Top with sesame seeds.
4) Finally, bake for 18 to 20 minutes. Allow it to cool completely and serve.

TAHINI PRALINE

Preparation Time: 5 Minutes | **Cooking Time**: 5 Minutes | **Servings**: Makes 15 Bars
Ingredients:
- 1 cup Tahini Paste
- 1 ½ cup Walnuts
- ½ cup Coconut Oil

Method of Preparation:
1) To start with, place the tahini butter, walnuts, and coconut oil in a large mixing bowl and combine them well until they are well combined.
2) Next, place the bowl in the freezer for about 1 to 1 ½ hours or until set.
3) Finally, slice them into small squares. Enjoy.

Tip: To make tahini paste, you need to take a cup of sesame seeds and toast them over medium-low heat for 5 minutes. Once the sesame seeds are cooled, place them in the food processor and process them for a minute or until you get a crumbly mixture. To this, pour the oil and salt. Process it again until you get a smooth paste.

ENERGY BALLS

Preparation Time: 10 Minutes | **Cooking Time: 10** Minutes | **Servings**: 1 Mason Jar
Ingredients:
- ¼ tsp. Salt
- ¾ cup Brazil Nuts; 2 tbsp. Coconut Oil
- ¾ cup Walnuts; ¼ cup of Dried Fruits
- ½ cup Sesame Seeds; ½ cup Hemp Hearts . ½ cup Figs, dried

Method of Preparation:
1) Begin by placing sesame seeds, salt, and figs in a food processor and process them for 2 to 3 minutes or until you get a sticky mixture. Transfer to a bowl.
2) After that, place the walnuts and brazil nuts in the processor and process until they are finely grounded yet crumbly in texture.
3) Then, add the walnut mixture to the sesame seeds mix. Combine.

4) Once combined, spoon in the dried fruits and hemp hearts. Mix and add the coconut. Combine again.
5) Finally, make rolls from the mixture and store it in an air-tight container.

Baked Kale Chips

Preparation Time: 10 Minutes
Cooking Time: 10 Minutes
Servings: 2 to 4
Ingredients:
- 1 lb. Kale, washed & patted dry
- Pure Sea Salt, as needed
- 1 tbsp. Grapeseed Oil
- Cayenne Pepper, as needed

Method of Preparation:
1) Preheat the oven to 350 ° F.
2) After that, tear off the kale leaves from the stem.
3) Now, place the kale leaves, grapeseed oil, sea salt and cayenne pepper in a large mixing bowl.
4) Massage the kale leaves with the seasoning and then place them on a parchment-paper-lined baking sheet.
5) Next, bake them for 8 minutes or until crispy.

Chips

Preparation Time: 10 Minutes | **Cooking Time:** 10 Minutes | **Servings**: 2 to 4
Ingredients:
- 1/3 cup Grapeseed Oil
- 2 cups Spelt Flour
- 1 tsp. Pure Sea Salt
- ½ cup Spring Water

Method of Preparation:
1) Preheat the oven to 350 ° F.
2) Next, place the spelt flour and the sea salt in the food processor and process it for 10 to 15 seconds.
3) After that, pour the grapeseed oil to it gradually while it is blending.
4) Continue blending until you get a smooth dough.
5) Then, place the dough on the floured work station.
6) Now, knead the dough for 2 minutes or until it becomes smooth.
7) Once it becomes smooth, keep the dough on a greased baking pan.
8) Apply oil and salt over the dough. Cut into triangles.
9) Finally, bake the triangles for 11 to 12 minutes or until they become golden brown in color.

DATES BALL

Preparation Time: 10 Minutes | **Cooking Time: 10** Minutes + 30 Minutes Marination Time
Servings: Makes 24 Balls
Ingredients:
- ½ cup Walnuts
- ½ tsp. Pure Sea Salt
- 1 cup Dates, pitted
- ¼ cup Agave Syrup
- 1 cup Coconut Meat
- ½ cup Sesame Seeds

Method of Preparation:
1) Begin by placing all the ingredients, excluding the sesame seeds in a high-speed blender and then pulse them 5 times for 20 seconds.
2) Then, transfer the mixture to a large plate.
3) Now, make balls out of it.
4) After that, dip them in the sesame coats and coat them thoroughly.
5) Serve and enjoy.

SWEETENED CHICKPEAS

Preparation Time: 5 Minutes | Cooking Time: 45 Minutes | **Servings**: Makes 1 cup
Ingredients:
- 15 oz. Garbanzo Beans, washed, drained & patted dry
- 2 tbsp. Agave Syrup
- ½ tsp. Pure Sea Salt
- 1 tbsp. Olive Oil

Method of Preparation:
1) Preheat the oven to 350 ° F.
2) After that, stir in the agave syrup, garbanzo beans, sea salt, and olive oil into a large mixing bowl and shake well.
3) Then, transfer the mixture to a parchment paper-lined baking tray and spread it across evenly in a single layer.
4) Finally, bake them for 45 minutes or until crispy.

RAISIN COOKIES

Preparation Time: 5 Minutes | Cooking Time: 45 Minutes | **Servings**: Makes 24 cookies
Ingredients:
- 2/3 cup Applesauce
- 1 cup Raisins
- 1 ½ cup Spelt Flour

- ½ tsp. Pure Sea Salt
- 1 ½ cup Spelt flakes, rolled
- 1/3 cup Grapeseed Oil
- 2 tbsp. Spring Water
- 1 ½ cup Dates, pitted
- 1/3 cup Agave

Method of Preparation:
1) For making these delicious cookies, you first need t to combine spelt flour, sea salt, and dates in a food processor.
2) Next, transfer the flour mix to a large mixing bowl and then add the spelt flakes to it.
3) After that, stir in all the remaining ingredients and give everything a good mix until you get a dough.
4) Now, make balls out of this dough and arrange them on a parchment paper-lined baking sheet.
5) Flatten the balls slightly with a fork.
6) Finally, bake them for 20 minutes at 350 °F.

Dr. Sebi

Desserts

Mango Coconut Sherbet

Preparation Time: 10 Minutes | **Cooking Time**: 5 Minutes | **Servings**: 4
Ingredients:
- 2 Mangoes, sweet
- ¼ cup Agave Nectar
- ½ cup Coconut Milk, raw

Method of Preparation:
1) For making this yummy sherbet, you need first to freeze the mangoes in the freezer for 8 hours.
2) Once frozen, blend them in the high-speed blender for 2 to 3 minutes or until smooth.
3) Next, stir in the coconut milk and agave nectar and blend again until you get a luxurious smooth sherbet.
4) Serve immediately.

Banana Walnut Ice Cream

Preparation Time: 10 Minutes | **Cooking Time**: 5 Minutes | **Servings**: 4
Ingredients:
- 1 cup Strawberries
- ½ of 1 Avocado, chopped
- ¼ cup Walnut Milk
- 5 Baby Bananas, quartered
- 1 tbsp. Agave Syrup

Method of Preparation:
1) Start by placing all the ingredients needed to make the ice cream in a high-speed blender for 2 minutes.
2) If it seems too thick, add more walnut milk.
3) Next, transfer the ice cream mixture to a large freezer-safe container and freeze them for 4 hours or until set.

Blueberry Chickpea Cake

Preparation Time: 10 Minutes | **Cooking Time**: 1 Hour | **Servings**: Makes 12 to 14 slices
Ingredients:
- 1 cup Garbanzo Flour
- Dash of Salt
- ¾ cup Spelt Flour
- 1 tbsp. Oil
- 1 cup Blueberries
- 6 tbsp. Agave Syrup
- ¾ cup Perrier
- 1 Clove, grounded

Method of Preparation:
1) To start with, place all the ingredients needed to make the cake in a high-speed blender and blend them on high speed for 4 to 5 minutes or until you get a smooth batter.
2) Next, transfer the batter to a parchment paper-lined baking pan and spread it evenly.
3) Now, bake the cake for 55 to 60 minutes or until cooked and the edges are slightly getting browned.

Walnut Date Nog

Preparation Time: 5 Minutes | Cooking Time: 5 Minutes **| Servings**: 2

Ingredients:
- ¼ cup Walnuts, chopped
- ½ tsp. Sea Salt
- 4 Dates, soaked
- 1 Clove, grounded
- 4 tbsp. Hemp Seeds
- Dash of Anise
- 2 tbsp. Agave Syrup
- 18 oz. Spring Water

Method of Preparation:
1) Start by placing all the ingredients needed to make the nog except clove and anise in a high-speed blender.
2) Blend for three minutes or until you get a smooth mixture.
3) Next, transfer the mixture to a medium-sized saucepan and warm the mixture.
4) Serve with a dash of clove and anise.
5) Enjoy.

Citrus Fruit Salad

Preparation Time: 10 Minutes | **Cooking Time: 10** Minutes + 30 Minutes Marination Time | **Servings**: 4

Ingredients:
- 8 oz. Grapes, seeded
- 1 Key Lime, quartered
- 8 Medjool Dates, sliced into halves
- 2 Kiwi, chopped
- 4 Seville Oranges, peeled & sliced

Method of Preparation:
1) To begin with, place all the ingredients needed to make the salad except the lime in a large mixing bowl.
2) Now, squeeze the lime all over the salad and toss well.
3) Serve and enjoy.

Mango Cheesecake

Preparation Time: 5 Minutes | **Cooking Time:** 4 Hour 30 Minutes | **Servings**: 8
Ingredients:
- 1 ½ cup Walnut Milk
- 2 cups Brazil Nuts
- ¼ tsp. Pure Sea Salt
- 6 Dates
- 2 tbsp. Lime Juice
- 1 tbsp. Sea Moss
- ¼ cup Agave Syrup

For the crust:
- 1/4 cup Agave Syrup
- ¼ tsp. Sea Salt
- 1 ½ cup Dates, quartered
- 1 ½ cup Coconut Flakes

Method of Preparation:
1) To begin with, place all the ingredients needed to make the crust in a food processor and process it for 30 to 45 minutes.
2) After that, place the crust mixture onto a parchment paper-lined baking sheet.
3) Now, spread out the mixture evenly across the sheet.
4) Then, spoon in the mango slices across the crust and place it in the freezer for 8 to 10 minutes.
5) Meanwhile, place all the filling ingredients in a high-speed blender. Blend until you get a smooth mixture.
6) Next, pour the filling mixture over the frozen crust and allow it to sit for 3 to 4 hours in the fridge.
7) Finally, before serving, garnish with more mango slices and strawberries.

Strawberry Sorbet

Preparation Time: 5 Minutes | **Cooking Time:** 10 Minutes + 4 Hours Chilling Time | **Servings**: 4
Ingredients:
- ½ cup Date Sugar
- 2 cups Strawberries
- 2 cups Spring Water
- 1 ½ tsp. Spelt Flour

Method of Preparation:
1) Begin by combing date sugar, spelt flour, and spring water in a medium-sized pot.
2) Next, heat the mixture over low heat and cook for 8 to 10 minutes or until thickened.
3) After that, take off the pot from the heat and allow it to cool.
4) Once cooled, puree the strawberries in a blender.

5) Now, mix the strawberry puree to the flour mixture and give everything a good stir.
6) Then, pour the mixture into a container and keep it in the freezer.
7) Cut the frozen sorbet to pieces and place it in the blender or food processor.
8) Blend until smooth and return the container to the refrigerator for a minimum of 4 hours.
9) Finally, serve the chilled strawberry sorbet.

STRAWBERRY ICE CREAM

Preparation Time: 5 Minutes | Cooking Time: 10 Minutes + 6 Hours Chilling Time **| Servings**: 3 to 4

Ingredients:
- ¼ cup Hemp Milk
- 1 cup Strawberries, frozen
- 1 tbsp. Agave Syrup
- 5 Baby Bananas, frozen
- ½ of 1 Avocado, ripe

Method of Preparation:
1) For making this delightful ice cream, place all the ingredients needed to make the ice cream in a high-speed blender.
2) Blend them for 2 to 3 minutes or until you get a smooth mixture.
3) Check for sweetness and add more agave syrup if needed.
4) Finally, transfer to a freezer-friendly container and freeze for at least 4 to 6 hours.

APPLESAUCE

Preparation Time: 5 Minutes | Cooking Time: 10 Minutes + 6 Hours Chilling Time **| Servings**: 4

Ingredients:
- 1 tsp. Sea Moss Gel
- 3 cups Apples, chopped
- 1/8 tsp. Pure Sea Salt
- 3 tbsp. Agave Syrup
- 1/8 tsp. Cloves
- 1 tsp. Lime Juice
- Spring Water, as needed

Method of Preparation:
1) First, keep all the ingredients needed to make the applesauce in the blender and blend for 3 minutes or until you get a smoothie with chunks in between.
2) Serve and enjoy.

Avocado Yoghurt Sauce

Preparation Time: 5 Minutes | Cooking Time: 5 Minutes **| Servings**: 2

Ingredients:
- 1/3 cup Agave Syrup
- 1 Avocado, ripe
- ¾ cup Spring Water
- Juice of 2 Limes
- 1 cup Berries

Method of Preparation:
1) Start by placing agave syrup, berries, lime juice, spring water, and avocado in a high-speed blender.
2) Blend them for 1 to 2 minutes or until smooth without any chunks.
3) Serve them cooled.

Dinner

SPELT BREAD

Preparation Time: 5 Minutes | **Cooking Time:** 70 Minutes | **Servings**: 4

Ingredients:
- 2 tsp. Pure Sea Salt
- 4 ½ cup Spelt Flour
- ¼ cup Agave Syrup
- 1 tsp. Sesame Seeds
- 2 tsp. Grape Seed Oil
- 2 cups Spring Water

Method of Preparation:
1) First, place the spelt flour and sea salt in a food processor for 10 to 20 seconds.
2) After that, stir in the agave syrup and mix well.
3) Then, spoon in the oil and water gradually to the mix until you get a dough.
4) Process the dough again for another 5 minutes.
5) Now, keep the dough in a greased & floured loaf pan.
6) Preheat the oven to 350 ° F. Allow it to sit for 1 hour.
7) Finally, bake it for 50 to 60 minutes or until cooked and browned.

CHAYOTE MUSHROOM SOUP

Preparation Time: 5 Minutes | **Cooking Time:** 10 Minutes | **Servings**: 8

Ingredients:
- 1 cup Hemp Milk; 1 tsp. Red Pepper, crushed
- 1 tbsp. Onion Powder
- 3 cups Mushroom, sliced
- 1 cup Onion, diced
- 2 cups Chayote Squash, cubed
- 2 tsp. Sea Salt
- 2 tsp. Basil; 2 tbsp. Grapeseed Oil
- 1 cup Vegetable Broth
- 1 ½ cup Garbanzo Flour
- 6 cups Spring Water

Method of Preparation:
1) First, place a deep saucepan over medium-high heat.
2) To this, spoon in the oil first, and once the oil becomes hot, stir in the mushrooms and onion. Then, add milk, seasonings, chayote, 4 cups of spring water and vegetable broth to it and cover it with a lid.
3) Next, transfer the mixture to a blender along with garbanzo flour and remaining water. Now, blend the mixture for 15 to 20 seconds or until they are no lumps.
4) Once blended, return the mixture to the pan and cook for 30 minutes while stirring it frequently. Serve it hot.

KALE WITH PEPPER

Preparation Time: 10 Minutes | **Cooking Time**: 15 Minutes | **Servings**: 4
Ingredients:
- ¼ cup Red Pepper, diced
- 1 bunch of kale, washed & pat dried
- 1 tsp. Grape Seed Oil
- ¼ cup Onion, diced
- ¼ tsp. Sea Salt
- 1 tsp. Chili, crushed

Method of Preparation:
1) To begin with, take the pat dried kale and fold each of them into a half. Slice off the stem.
2) Next, tear the leaves into smaller pieces. After that, spoon the oil into a wok over high heat.
3) To this, stir in the onion and pepper along with salt. Cook for 3 minutes and reduce the heat to low. Now, add the kale to the wok and cook for another 5 minutes while keeping it covered. Then, stir in the crushed red pepper and give everything a good stir.
4) Cook for another 3 minutes or until tender.
5) Remove from heat and serve immediately.

ZUCCHINI PASTA

Preparation Time: 10 Minutes | **Cooking Time**: 15 Minutes | **Servings**: 2 to 3
Ingredients:
- 4 Zucchini, large & spiralized
- ¼ tsp. Sea Salt
- 2 Avocadoes, medium
- 2 tbsp. Grapeseed Oil
- 1 cup Cherry Tomatoes
- ¼ cup Basil, fresh

Method of Preparation:
1) First, spiralize the zucchini with a spiralizer or make thin strips using a vegetable peeler.
2) After that, spoon oil into a large skillet over medium heat.
3) To this, stir in the zoodles and cook them for 4 to 5 minutes or until tender and cooked.
4) Remove from heat. Transfer to a large serving bowl.
5) Now, stir in the cherry tomatoes, avocadoes, salt, and basil.
6) Toss well and serve.

CHICKPEAS CORNBREAD

Preparation Time: 10 Minutes | **Cooking Time**: 15 Minutes | **Servings**: Makes 14 squares
Ingredients:
- 2 cup Chickpea Flour
- 1 cup Brazil Nut Milk
- 1 cup Applesauce
- Water, as needed
- ½ cup Grapeseed Oil

- 1 tbsp. Pepper

Method of Preparation:
1) To start with, combine all the ingredients needed to make the cornbread in a large mixing bowl until it is smooth. It should be of medium consistency.
2) After that, if the batter seems too thickened, you can use water to thin it out.
3) Now, brush the pan with the grapeseed oil and then pour the batter into it. Spread it out evenly. Bake for 28 to 30 minutes or until a toothpick inserted in the center comes clean.
4) Once cooled, slice into squares.

ZUCCHINI BREAD

Preparation Time: 10 Minutes | **Cooking Time**: 40 Minutes | **Servings**: 3 to 4
Ingredients:
- 2 tbsp. Oil
- 1 cup Zucchini Puree
- 1 cup Spelt Flour
- Dash of Salt
- 1 tbsp. Perrier

Method of Preparation:
1) First, mix the zucchini puree with the spelt flour, oil, salt, and Perrier in a large mixing bowl until everything comes together.
2) To this, pour more water as needed to get a thick yet smooth dough.
3) Now, spread the dough into a greased parchment paper-lined baking sheet.
4) Bake for 33 minutes at 350 ° F or until cooked.

CHICKPEA SOUP

Preparation Time: 5 Minutes
Cooking Time: 5 Minutes
Servings: 2 to 3
Ingredients:
- 2 cups Chickpeas
- ½ tsp. Cayenne Pepper
- 1 Zucchini, small
- Spring Water, as needed
- 1 Bell Pepper, diced
- 1 Onion, small & diced

Method of Preparation:
1) To start with, spoon some oil and then place all the ingredients needed to make the soup in a deep saucepan over medium heat.
2) Cook the ingredients for 7 minutes or until cooked and al dente.
3) Now, cool the veggies slightly and then transfer them to a high-speed blender and blend for 2 to 3 minutes or until smooth. Serve and enjoy.

Dr. Sebi

STRAWBERRY SALAD

Preparation Time: 5 Minutes | **Cooking Time:** 5 Minutes | **Servings**: 2 to 3
Ingredients:
- 2 tbsp. Grapeseed Oil
- 10 Strawberries, sliced
- 1 Red Onion, sliced
- Pure Sea Salt, as needed
- 4 cups Dandelion Greens, washed and torn
- 2 tbsp. Key Lime Juice
- 1 tbsp. Sesame Seeds
- Pure Sea Salt, as needed

Method of Preparation:
1) Heat a large saucepan over medium-high heat.
2) Once the pan becomes hot, spoon in the oil.
3) Next, sprinkle the salt over the red onion slices.
4) Then, stir the onion slices onto it.
5) Cook the salted onion for 2 minutes or until softened.
6) Now, spoon one tablespoon of lime juice over it and continue cooking for another 2 minutes. After that, spoon the remaining lime juice over the strawberries in a large mixing bowl.
7) Finally, add the dandelion greens into the bowl along with the sautéed onions.
8) Sprinkle the sesame seeds and pure sea salt over it and toss well.
9) Serve immediately.

MASHED SQUASH

Preparation Time: 5 Minutes | **Cooking Time:** 5 Minutes | **Servings**: 6
Ingredients:
- 1 tsp. Allspice
- ¼ cup Blue Agave, organic
- 2 Squash, peeled & cut into chunks
- 1/8 tsp. Pure Sea Salt
- ¼ cup Date Sugar
- ¼ cup Hemp Milk

Method of Preparation:
1) To start with, place the squash chunks along with spring water in a pot over medium heat.
2) Bring the mixture to a boil and cook for 20 minutes or until the squash becomes tender. Once tender, drain away the water and mash the squash.
3) To this, spoon in the date sugar, sea salt, all spice, hemp milk and agave. Mix well.
4) Serve and enjoy it.

Quinoa Avocado Salad

Preparation Time: 5 Minutes | **Cooking Time:** 5 Minutes | **Servings**: 2

Ingredients:
- 1 cup Quinoa
- 14 oz. Chickpeas, drained
- 1 Avocado, ripe & quartered
- Basil, fresh & torn to pieces

Method of Preparation:
1) Start by cooking the quinoa by following the instructions given on the package.
2) Once cooked, transfer the quinoa to a large mixing bowl.
3) Next, stir in the remaining ingredients and give a good stir.
4) Check for seasoning and add more salt if needed.
5) Serve with lime wedges and drizzle oil over it if desired.

Macaroni & Cheese

Preparation Time: 5 Minutes | **Cooking Time:** 10 Minutes | **Servings**: 8 to 10

Ingredients:
- 1 cup Hemp Milk
- 12 oz. Kamut Pasta
- 1 tsp. Pure Sea Salt
- ½ tsp. All Spice
- ¼ cup Garbanzo Bean Flour
- ½ lb. Brazil Nuts, raw & soaked
- Juice of ½ of 1 Lime
- 1 cup Spring Water
- 2 tsp. Onion Powder
- 2 tsp. Grapeseed Oil

Method of Preparation:
1) For making this healthy fare, cook the pasta by following the instructions given on the packet.
2) After that, preheat the oven to 350 °F.
3) Then, place all the ingredients needed to make the dressing in a high-speed blender.
4) Blend for 2 minutes or until everything becomes smooth.
5) Now, heat the oil in a large skillet over medium-high heat.
6) Once the oil becomes hot, stir in the pasta and sauté for 1 minute.
7) Next, pour the sauce to the skillet and give everything a good stir.
8) Finally, bake the pasta for 30 minutes or until cooked.

SAUTÉED GREENS

Preparation Time: 5 Minutes | **Cooking Time:** 10 Minutes | **Servings:** 8 to 10
Ingredients:
- 3 bunches of Turnip Green
- 3 tbsp. Pure Sea Salt
- 2 cups Onions, chopped
- 1 tsp. Cayenne Pepper
- 1 tbsp. Olive Oil

Method of Preparation:
1) To start with, sauté the onions in a medium-sized skillet over medium heat.
2) Once cooked, stir in the greens and cook for 18 to 20 minutes.
3) Finally, season it with salt and cayenne pepper.

VEGGIE QUINOA

Preparation Time: 5 Minutes | **Cooking Time:** 10 Minutes | **Servings:** 6 to 8
Ingredients:
- 1 tsp. Basil
- 4 cups Quinoa, cooked
- 1 tsp. Oregano
- 1 cup Zucchini, chopped
- 2 tsp. Pure Sea Salt
- ¼ cup Red Bell Pepper, chopped
- ½ cup Onion, diced
- ¼ cup Green Bell Pepper, chopped
- ½ tsp. Cayenne Pepper
- ¼ cup Yellow Bell Pepper, chopped
- 1 Plum Tomato, chopped
- ½ cup Spring Water
- 1 tbsp. Onion Powder
- 2 tbsp. Grapeseed Oil

Method of Preparation:
1) First, spoon oil to a large frying pan over medium heat.
2) Then, stir in the veggies and seasoning to it and cook for further 5 minutes or until tender.
3) Now, pour the water along with the quinoa to it.
4) Give everything a good stir and continue cooking for another 2 minutes.
5) Serve it hot.

Dips & Sauces

MAYONNAISE

Preparation Time: 5 Minutes | **Cooking Time:** 5 Minutes | **Servings**: 1 Mason Jar
Ingredients:
- 1 tsp. Sea Salt
- 3 tbsp. Coconut Oil; 1 tbsp. Onion Powder
- Juice from ½ of 1 Key Lime; 1 tsp. Salt

Method of Preparation:
1) Start by placing all the ingredients needed to make the mayonnaise in a high-speed blender for 2 to 3 minutes or until you get a smooth mixture.
2) Store in an air-tight container.

MANGO SALSA

Preparation Time: 5 Minutes | **Cooking Time: 5** Minutes | **Servings**: 3 cups
Ingredients:
- 6 Plum Tomatoes ; ½ tsp. Cayenne Pepper
- 1 Tomatillo; 1 tsp. Sea Salt
- ½ cup Red Onion, chopped; 1 tsp. Onion Powder
- ¼ cup Green Bell Pepper; ½ cup Cilantro
- ½ cup Mango, chopped; Juice from ½ of 1 Lemon

Method of Preparation:
1) First, combine all the ingredients needed to make the salsa, excluding the mango in the food processor. Process them 10 to 15 seconds and then add the mango to it.
2) Scrape the sides and blend well for another 20 seconds.
3) Transfer to a bowl and enjoy.

GUACAMOLE

Preparation Time: 5 Minutes | **Cooking Time:** 5 Minutes | **Servings**: 2 ½ cups
Ingredients:
- 2 Avocadoes, halved
- ½ cup Cilantro, chopped; 1 Plum Tomato, diced
- Juice of ½ of 1 Lime ; ½ cup Onion, diced
- ½ tsp. Sea Salt; ½ tsp. Cayenne Powder

Method of Preparation:
1) Start by slicing the avocadoes into halves and then scoop out the flesh into a bowl.
2) After that, stir in all the remaining ingredients into it, excluding the plum tomato.
3) Mix them well by using a masher.
4) Next, spoon in the diced tomatoes and combine them again.

CUCUMBER DRESSING

Preparation Time: 5 Minutes | **Cooking Time:** 5 Minutes | **Servings**: 2 ½ cups
Ingredients:
- 1 cup Cucumber, quartered
- ¼ cup Avocado Oil
- 1 tsp. Dill, fresh
- 1 tbsp. Lime Juice
- ½ tsp. Onion Powder
- 2 tsp. Agave Syrup

Method of Preparation:
1) To begin with, place all the ingredients needed to make the dressing in a high-speed blender.
2) Blend for two minutes or until you get a smooth paste.

SALSA VERDE

Preparation Time: 5 Minutes | Cooking Time: 5 Minutes |**Servings**: Makes 2 cup
Ingredients:
- ¼ cup Cilantro
- 1 tsp. Onion Powder
- 1 lb. Tomatillo, washed, skin removed & halved
- 1 tsp. Pure Sea Salt
- ½ cup Onion, diced; 1 tsp. Oregano

Method of Preparation:
1) For making this yummy dip, place the onions along with other ingredients, excluding the cilantro in a saucepan over medium heat. Fill it with water.
2) Now, cook the mixture for 20 minutes while stirring it occasionally.
3) Then, pour the juice through a strainer to a bowl, and to this, add the cilantro.
4) Next, transfer the mixture to a high-speed blender and blend for half a minute.

AVOCADO SAUCE

Preparation Time: 5 Minutes |**Cooking Time: 5** Minutes |**Servings**: Makes 1 cup
Ingredients:
- ½ tsp. Oregano
- ½ tsp. Pure Sea Salt
- 1 Avocado, pitted
- 2 tbsp. Onion, chopped
- ½ tsp. Onion Powder; Dash of Basil, chopped

Method of Preparation:
1) First, place the avocado meat to the high-speed blender along with the remaining ingredients. Blend the mixture for 3 minutes or until everything becomes smooth without any lumps.

Hummus

Preparation Time: 5 Minutes | Cooking Time: 10 Minutes | Servings: Makes 1 cup

Ingredients:
- 2 tbsp. Olive Oil
- 1/3 cup Tahini Paste
- 2 tbsp. Key Lime Juice
- 1 cup Garbanzo Beans, cooked
- Pure Sea Salt, as needed; ½ tsp. Onion Powder

Method of Preparation:
1) Start by placing all the ingredients required to make the hummus in a food processor and process them for 2 to 3 minutes or until you get a creamy paste.

BBQ Sauce

Preparation Time: 5 Minutes | Cooking Time: 40 Minutes | Servings: Makes 1 cup

Ingredients:
- 1/8 tsp. Cloves
- 6 Plum Tomatoes, quartered
- 2 tsp. Pure Sea Salt
- ¼ cup Onion, chopped
- 2 tsp. Onion Powder
- ¼ tsp. Cayenne
- ¼ cup Date Sugar
- 2 tbsp. Agave Syrup

Method of Preparation:
1) To begin with, place all the ingredients needed to make the sauce in a high-speed blender.
2) Blend them for 1 to 2 minutes or until you get a smooth paste.
3) Now, transfer the mixture to a medium-sized saucepan and to this, stir in the date sugar.
4) Cook over medium heat while stirring it frequently.
5) Next, reduce the heat to low and allow it to simmer for 10 to 15 minutes while covering it with a lid. Stir frequently.
6) Then with an immersion blender, blend it again until smooth.
7) Return the sauce back to the saucepan and cook for further 10 minutes.
8) Allow it to cool and then store.

Mango Dressing

Preparation Time: 5 Minutes | Cooking Time: 10 Minutes | Servings: Makes ½ cup

Ingredients:
- 1/4 tsp. Pure Sea Salt

Dr. Sebi

- 1 cup Mango, chopped
- 1 tsp. Onion Powder
- 2 tbsp. Key Lime Juice
- 1 tsp. Basil
- ¼ cup Grape Seed Oil
- 1 tsp. Agave Syrup

Method of Preparation:
1) First, place all the ingredients needed to make the sauce in a high-speed blender.
2) Blend for 1 to 2 minutes or until you get a smooth paste.

TOMATO SAUCE

Preparation Time: 5 Minutes | Cooking Time: 40 Minutes | Servings: Makes 6 cup
Ingredients:

- 3 tsp. Basil
- 1/8 tsp. Cayenne Pepper
- 18 Roma Tomatoes, halved
- 3 tsp. Basil
- ½ of 1 Sweet Onion, halved
- 2 tsp. Onion Powder
- ½ of 1 Red Onion, halved
- ½ of 1 Bell Pepper, diced & halved
- 1 tbsp. Agave Syrup
- 2 tsp. Oregano
- 3 tsp. Pure Sea Salt
- 1/8 cup Grapeseed Oil

Method of Preparation:
1) Preheat the oven to 400 ° F.
2) After that, place the vegetables in the large mixing bowl.
3) To this, pour one teaspoon of grapeseed oil along with sea salt and basil. Toss well.
4) Now, arrange the coated vegetables in a greased baking sheet.
5) Then, roast the veggies for 25 to 30 minutes. Turn the sheet halfway.
6) Once the veggies are roasted, place them in the blender and blend them for 1 minute or until you get a smooth paste.
7) Finally, transfer the mixture to a medium-sized pot over medium heat and cook for further 20 minutes.
8) Serve and enjoy it.

COLESLAW

Preparation Time: 5 Minutes
Cooking Time: 40 Minutes
Servings: 4
Ingredients:

- ½ tsp. Sea Moss Gel
- 2 cups Zucchini, shredded
- ½ cup Springwater
- ½ tsp. Lime Juice
- ½ cup Brazil nuts
- ¼ cups Onion, diced
- ½ cup Spring Water
- ½ tsp. Lime Juice
- ¼ cup Hemp Milk
- ¼ tsp. Dates, spammed

Method of Preparation
1) To start with, place all the ingredients needed to make excluding the veggies in a food processor and blend for 2 to 3 minutes or until
2) Then transfer the mixture to a plate.
3) In the meantime, cook the veggies.
4) Once all the veggies are cooked, shake the container.

Hot Sauce

Preparation Time: 5 Minutes
Cooking Time: 30 Minutes
Servings: Makes 1 cup
Ingredients:
- 1 tbsp. Sea Moss Powder
- 1 ½ cups Spring Water
- 2 tbsp. Onion Powder
- ½ cup Key Lime Juice
- 2 tbsp. Cayenne Pepper
- 9 Plum Tomatoes
- ½ tsp. Pure Sea Salt

Method of Preparation
1) Begin by placing all the ingredients needed to make the hot sauce in a high-speed blender and blend them for 3 minutes or until you get a smooth paste.
2) After that, heat the mixture in a deep saucepan over medium-high heat.
3) Cook the mixture for 10 to 15 minutes and then allow it to cool slightly.
4) Store in an air-tight container.

Smoothies

STRAWBERRY BANANA SMOOTHIE

Preparation Time: 5 Minutes | **Cooking Time**: 5 Minutes | **Servings**: 1 to 2
Ingredients:
- 2 cups Hemp Milk
- 4 Banana
- 8 oz. Strawberry
- ¾ cup Dates
- 1 tbsp. Agave

Method of Preparation:
1) For making this delicious smoothie, you need to place the strawberries and date in a high-speed blender.
2) Blend them for a minute or two or until slightly broken down.
3) After that, add the banana along with the hemp milk and agave.
4) Blend them for 2 to 3 minutes or until combined well.
5) Enjoy.

GREEN MONSTER SMOOTHIE

Preparation Time: 5 Minutes | **Cooking Time**: 5 Minutes | **Servings**: 1
Ingredients:
- ½ of 1 Avocado, diced
- ½ of 1 Mango, diced
- 2 to 3 Dates, pitted
- 1 tbsp. Soursop Pulp
- 1 Bunch of Rainbow Kale, leaves torn
- ½ cup Coconut Water

Method of Preparation:
1) For making this smoothie, place all the ingredients in a high-speed blender and blend it for 2 to 3 minutes or until everything comes together and smooth.
2) Transfer the mixture to a serving glass and serve it with ice cubes if you desire to take it cold.

Cucumber Coconut Smoothie

Preparation Time: 5 Minutes
Cooking Time: 5 Minutes
Servings: 1
Ingredients:
- 2 Cucumbers
- 1 tsp. Agave Nectar
- 1 Young Coconut
- 1-inch Ginger

Method of Preparation:
1) First, place all the ingredients in a large bowl and combine well until everything comes together.
2) Serve cold or warm.

Apple Smoothie

Preparation Time: 5 Minutes
Cooking Time: 20 Minutes
Servings: 2
Ingredients:
- 1 tbsp. Sea Moss
- 2 cups Ice
- 2 cups Apple Juice, fresh
- 1 tbsp. Ginger
- Dash of Clove Powder

Method of Preparation:
1) For making this delicious smoothie, place all the ingredients needed to make the smoothie in a high-speed blender.
2) Blend for 1 ½ minute or until you get a creamy smoothie.
3) Now, stir in the ice and blend for further one minute.
4) Finally, transfer to a serving glass and enjoy it.

BERRY WALNUT SMOOTHIE

Preparation Time: 5 Minutes
Cooking Time: 5 Minutes
Servings: 2
Ingredients:
- 1 cup Walnuts, raw & soaked for 8 hours
- ½ cup Coconut Milk
- 2 Figs, soaked for 8 hours
- 1 tbsp. Key Lime Juice
- ¼ cup Strawberries
- 1 tsp. Agave Syrup

Method of Preparation:
1) For making this tasty smoothie, place all the ingredients needed to make the smoothie in a high-speed blender.
2) Blend for 3 minutes or until smooth.
3) Transfer to a serving glass and top it with nuts approved by dr. Sebi.

WATERMELON SMOOTHIE

Preparation Time: 5 Minutes
Cooking Time: 5 Minutes
Servings: 1
Ingredients:
- 1 cup Coconut Water
- 1 cup Watermelon Pieces
- 1 tbsp. Date Syrup
- 1 cup Strawberries

Method of Preparation:
1) Begin by blending watermelon, strawberries, coconut water, and date syrup in a high-speed blender for 1 to 2 minutes or until smooth and rich.
2) Transfer to a serving glass and enjoy it.

Peach Berry Smoothie

Preparation Time: 5 Minutes | Cooking Time: 5 Minutes | Servings: 1

Ingredients:
- 1 tbsp. Sea Moss
- 1 cup Coconut Milk
- ½ cup Strawberries
- 1 tbsp. Hemp Seeds
- ½ cup Peaches, quartered
- 1 tbsp. Agave Syrup
- ½ cup Blueberries

Method of Preparation:
1) First, keep strawberries, agave syrup, sea moss, hemp seeds, coconut milk, blueberries, peaches, and blueberries in the high-speed blender.
2) Blend for 1 minute or until you get a smooth and luxurious smoothie.
3) Transfer to a serving glass and serve immediately. Enjoy.

Cucumber Tomato Smoothie

Preparation Time: 5 Minutes | Cooking Time: 5 Minutes | Servings: 1

Ingredients:
- 1 Cucumber
- 3 tbsp. Agave Syrup
- 1 Plum Tomato
- 2 cups Water

Method of Preparation:
1) For making this healthy smoothie, place all the ingredients needed to make the smoothie in a high-speed blender or until smooth.
2) Next, transfer to a large serving glass and enjoy it.

Detox Green Smoothie

Preparation Time: 5 Minutes | Cooking Time: 5 Minutes | Servings: 1

Ingredients:
- 2 cups Amaranth Greens
- 2 cups Water
- 1 Key Lime
- 2 Apples, cored
- ¼ of 1 Avocado, cubed

Method of Preparation:
1) First, place greens, apple, avocado, key lime, and water in a high-speed blender and blend for 1 to 1 ½ minute or until you get a rich and creamy smoothie.
2) Serve and enjoy.

PEAR SMOOTHIE

Preparation Time: 5 Minutes | **Cooking Time:** 5 Minutes | **Servings**: 1
Ingredients:
- ¼ cup Quinoa, cooked
- 1 Pear, chopped
- 1 oz. Blueberries
- ¼ of 1 Avocado, pitted
- 1 cup Water

Method of Preparation:
1) Start by placing all the ingredients needed to make the smoothie in a high-speed blender.
2) Blend for 2 minutes or until you get a thick smoothie.

CUCUMBER WATERMELON SMOOTHIE

Preparation Time: 5 Minutes | **Cooking Time:** 5 Minutes | **Servings**: 1
Ingredients:
- 1 Cucumber
- 1 cup Watermelon, cubed
- 1 Key Lime

Method of Preparation:
1) First, place the cucumber, watermelon, and key lime in a high-speed blender for 1 to 2 minutes or until you get a smooth mixture.
2) Now, transfer to a serving glass and enjoy it.

ORANGE BERRY SMOOTHIE

Preparation Time: 5 Minutes | **Cooking Time:** 5 Minutes | **Servings**: 1
Ingredients:
- 1 Burro Banana, medium
- 1 cup Berries
- 1 Seville Orange
- ¼ of 1 Avocado, ripe
- 2 cups Lettuce, fresh
- Spring Water, as needed
- 1 tbsp. Hemp Seeds

Method of Preparation:
1) For making this delicious smoothie, blend all the ingredients in a high-speed blender for 2 to 3 minutes or until you get a rich and luscious smoothie.

Banana Ginger Smoothie

Preparation Time: 5 Minutes | Cooking Time: 5 Minutes **| Servings**: 1
Ingredients:
- 1 Banana, frozen
- 1 tbsp. Agave Syrup
- 2 cups Hemp Milk
- ½ cup Strawberries, chopped
- 1 handful of Kale
- 1-inch piece of Ginger, minced finely

Method of Preparation:
1) Start by blending all the ingredients in a high-speed blender for 3 minutes or until you get a luscious smoothie without any chunks.
2) Serve immediately and enjoy it.

Papaya Smoothie

Preparation Time: 5 Minutes | Cooking Time: 5 Minutes **| Servings**: 1
Ingredients:
- ½ cup Coconut Milk
- 1 cup Papaya
- 1 tsp. Lime Juice
- 4 Strawberries
- ½ cup Pineapple, frozen
- ¼-inch Ginger

Method of Preparation:
1) To begin with, place all the ingredients needed to make the papaya smoothie in a high-speed blender for 2 minutes.
2) Once it becomes smooth and luscious, transfer to a serving glass.

Quinoa Pear Smoothie

Preparation Time: 5 Minutes | Cooking Time: 5 Minutes **| Servings**: 1
Ingredients:
- ¼ of 1 Avocado, pitted
- 1 cup Water
- ¼ cup Quinoa, cooked
- 1 cup Spring Water
- 1 oz. Blueberries
- 1 Pear

Method of Preparation:
1) First, mix all the ingredients needed to make the smoothie in a high-speed blender for 3 minutes or until smooth and creamy.
2) Transfer to a glass and enjoy it.

Made in the USA
San Bernardino, CA
07 March 2020